THE ULTIMATE PREGNANCY SURVIVAL GUIDE FOR FIRST-TIME DADS

A COMPREHENSIVE GUIDE FOR SUPPORTING YOUR PARTNER, BONDING WITH YOUR BABY, AND BECOMING A CONFIDENT FATHER

PATRICK NGUYEN

CONTENTS

INTRODUCTION

Picture this: I'm sitting in the doctor's office, anxiously tapping my foot on the linoleum floor. My heart is racing, and my mind is filled with a whirlwind of emotions. My wife is sitting beside me, her hand tightly gripping mine. We've been waiting for what feels like an eternity to hear the pregnancy test results. Seconds turn into minutes, and the suspense is unbearable. Then, the doctor walks in, a knowing smile on his face, as he says those magical words, *"Congratulations, you're going to be a dad!"*

At that moment, my entire world shifted. The positive home pregnancy test caused an emotional roller coaster. But this was a whole new level of anxiety and excitement. The doctor's confirmation resounded in my head as the fearsome weight of responsibility, excitement, and pure awe settled on my shoulders. It was as if a switch had been flipped, and I knew that life as I knew it would never be the same again. I realized this was all too real and that I suddenly embarked on an incredible journey into fatherhood filled with joy, challenges, and many surprises.

But all along, my steps were hounded by feelings of fear, expectation and uncertainty, worry and anxiousness. Yet, deep down, I knew these feelings were normal. So I tried to stand tall and tough. I attempted to prepare for whatever was coming. But men can never fully ready themselves to be the most supportive partners and caring fathers. We can only do our best.

Now, if you're reading this, chances are you've experienced a similar moment - the moment you discovered that you were going to be a father. And more than likely, you are feeling those same emotions and feelings. But let me tell you, my friend, you're in for an extraordinary ride. The next nine months will be a whirlwind of emotions, revelations, and incredible, rewarding growth. But fear not! You hold in your hands the ultimate survival guide that will equip you with everything you need to know about pregnancy, birth, and beyond, explicitly tailored for first-time dads like you.

This is not just another run-of-the-mill parenting book. It's a roadmap, a companion, and a lifeline, all rolled into one. Together, we will navigate the uncharted territory of each trimester of pregnancy, childbirth, and early fatherhood. I will share with you the wisdom I gained from my own experiences and those of fellow fathers who have walked this path before us.

In the following chapters, we will dive deep into the physical and emotional changes your partner experiences during pregnancy. We'll explore the mysteries of prenatal care, childbirth classes, and creating a supportive environment at home. Likewise, we will discuss the common concerns and fears that might keep you up at night, and together we will reveal the secrets to being the unshakable rock that your partner needs during this transformative time.

But this guide isn't just about the technicalities of pregnancy. It's about embracing your role as an equal partner and an engaged provider. We'll talk about the importance of fostering open communication with your partner, nurturing a solid foundation of love and respect, and navigating the delicate balance between work and family life. We'll delve into the magic of bonding with your baby, the challenges of sleep deprivation, and the joy of witnessing your child's first milestones.

Throughout this book, you'll find a wealth of knowledge, expert insights, and heartwarming examples to make you laugh, cry, or nod your head in recognition. We'll tackle the tough questions, address the doubts that may linger in your mind, and celebrate the victories, no matter how small. Because, my friend, you're not alone on this journey. Countless dads have gone before you, and countless more will come after. Together, we form a brotherhood - a tribe of fathers navigating the beautiful chaos of fatherhood, all for you to become the involved partner and confident father you wish to be.

Aside from its in-depth and refreshing take on pregnancy and fatherhood, this book will also help you A.C.E. this period of your life by inviting you to assess, center in, and embrace the ups and downs of being a dad. Our unique A.C.E. method (Awareness, Connection, Embrace) tackles the age-old fatherhood questions in a new, innovative, and super-efficient manner that will completely revolutionize how you experience and thrive during your partner's pregnancy.

And best of all, you'll be getting useful, first-hand information. Because, after all, who better to share the secrets of fatherhood - than an experienced father? As a devoted husband, a hard-working provider, and a proud father of three, I will share with you all the knowledge I accumulated, along with expert recommendations from various medical resources.

With my background as a registered nurse, it's my duty. I am providing first-time dads the ultimate guide that I didn't have during my wife's first pregnancy. Many years later, I realized how such a handy guidebook could have helped me become a more supportive partner and a confident father-to-be from the beginning. DISCLAIMER: This book is not meant to replace medical advice. Please consult your healthcare providers with your concerns.

So, as we embark on this adventure together, I invite you to open your heart, embrace the unknown, and prepare to be amazed. This book is here to support, inspire, and empower you as you become the confident father you were destined to be. With just a bit of hard work, you, too, can become a caring partner, a wonderful father, and an exemplary role model for other expectant fathers. And in the end, you will sit back and think that, after all, first-time fatherhood wasn't as difficult as you thought it would be. So let's dive in and embrace this incredible dad journey, one page at a time.

1

LET'S CLEAR THE AIR

S o, congratulations are in order! You have embarked on a monumental nine-month journey with your partner that will be transformative, rewarding, and - in many ways - life-changing. Happiness awaits you in the end, but there will be many challenges to overcome. Still, the pregnancy journey is unique to every person and every couple. It would be best if you didn't take every bit of information as a definitive statement and something that *has* to happen to you. That, you have to agree, would be silly.

Still, we understand your feelings. This is a big thing, after all - a life-changing thing - and you want to do everything to be fully prepared for what's coming. As a first-time father, you can be assaulted by a flurry of myths, preconceptions, and old-wives'-tales that can create unnecessary fear and anxiety. It is crucial to separate fact from fiction and debunk these common pregnancy myths to provide expectant fathers with accurate information and peace of mind.

We're here to dispel these myths, eradicate them, and set the actual facts in stone - once and for all. Together, we will shed light on the truth behind these misconceptions, promoting a better understanding of this beautiful phase of life.

Once the realization settles in and you finally embrace the fact that you will be a father to a tiny baby boy or girl, your mind enters an entirely different mindset of preparation. You want to do everything to be ready when the time comes and be the best parent you can be. But if you are faced with misconceptions or lack guidance, you may quickly embrace any old rumor you hear. That can only make the expectations worse.

But if you begin your journey one step at a time, composed and calm, you can decipher fact from fiction and prepare yourself correctly.

COMMON PREGNANCY MYTHS

Now, which is the right way? You could be showered with conflicting advice from every side: your parents will offer popular tips from their generation; every doctor will have their own point of view; and the internet will be chocked full of random information and opinions. In no time, you can be flooded with tips that are nothing more than common myths. Here are just some common pregnancy-related myths that *always* get thrown around:

- **Pregnant women *need* to eat for two.**

While it is undoubtedly true that the number of calories an expecting mother should consume during the day will have to increase slightly, it does not mean she should start overeating. Such a massive increase in caloric intake can do more harm than good. Suppose your partner is already consuming a regular diet. In that case, a moderate, simple increase in calories is all that is required. Of course, it is more important for the woman to start consuming a balanced and healthy diet without any bad calories, alcohol, or nicotine. Those old wives' tales of eating like there's no tomorrow, pickle cravings, and similar myths are ready to be busted.

- **Your partner should steer clear from exercise during pregnancy.**

This misconception causes many divisions in the scientific and medical circles. Should a pregnant woman engage in physical exercise during pregnancy? Some old-school doctors and most grandmas will staunchly state that activity of any kind is harmful. According to them, it's all about rest, rest, rest. But it might be more complex. Many modern doctors suggest light to moderate aerobic exercise in the first trimester, about 2 to 5 times per week. Women that haven't been engaging in any physical activity before pregnancy are not advised to start during this time. However, women who exercise regularly may continue light exercise during the first stages of pregnancy and have higher chances of a smoother, easier delivery.

- **Women should avoid sexual intercourse during pregnancy.**

This is a myth that every expecting couple wants to figure out. Is sex harmful in pregnancy? The truth is - *no*, sex has no detrimental effect on a normal pregnancy. And no, you will not be poking at your baby's head. Sex actually has its benefits! You can improve your intimacy and bond as a couple and reduce your and your partner's stress levels. Another advantage is that you can strengthen your partner's pelvic floor. It is common for women to struggle with incontinence after birth, which is the inability to hold in their pee when they have to use the bathroom. Strengthening the pelvic floor by having sex during pregnancy can help prevent that issue. Lastly, sex can induce labor by helping your partner produce contractions. Remember this for the third trimester, near your baby's due date. Of course, suppose something is out of the ordinary. In that case, your doctor can advise that you abstain from intercourse for specific periods. But if everything is normal, then don't be afraid to get intimate with your partner!

- **Caffeine is off-limits for pregnant women.**

Everyone loves a cup of coffee in the morning or an espresso shot in the afternoon. But is it the same for pregnant women? Modern research shows that women can still enjoy coffee during pregnancy, albeit in moderate amounts. One to one and a half cups of coffee per day is allowed. This equals about 200mg of caffeine daily, considering a cup is 8 ounces. Anything above this is not advised.

- **You can accurately predict the sex of your baby.**

For the most part, this myth is totally false. No matter what you do, you can't predict the baby's gender without doing particular tests such as an ultrasound, a blood test, or an amniotic fluid test. Many popular tales exist, such as observing the shape of the woman's belly, the things she craves, how she behaves, or the quality of her skin during pregnancy. Needless to say, these things are unrelated to your baby's sex.

- **When you're over 35, pregnancy is dangerous.**

If your partner happens to be over 35, you could see her pregnancy labeled as "high risk." From this appeared a popular myth related to pregnancies after you're 35. The "high risk" label comes simply because certain risks are just a tad bit higher at that age. It does *not* mean that they are inevitable and sure to happen. Women in their late 30s and 40s can experience normal pregnancies and standard deliveries and bring healthy and happy babies into the world. Another myth debunked!

- **Breastfeeding is a simple, natural thing.**

Many first-time parents will think that breastfeeding is a thing that "nature takes care of" - i.e., it's a matter of instincts that kick in when the baby comes. While there is certainly truth to this, it can sometimes be complicated. Sometimes, it is a challenging process. It can take time to find the ideal positioning for the baby to latch onto the nipple, establish a routine of frequent feedings, and for mild production to truly kick into full gear. It is perfectly normal for you and your partner to seek help and coaching with breastfeeding and lactation.

- **Pregnancy creates all sorts of weird cravings.**

We all know that classic stereotype: pregnant women *crave* odd foods such as pickles, ice cream, or anything in between. This is just another popular myth. Of course, women might crave specific foods or beverages during pregnancy, but there aren't any rules to this. Usually, it is a way for a woman's body to acquire the specific nutrients it needs. Personally, my wife craved ice cream in the middle of the night. Her body might have been telling her she needed more calories from not eating due to nausea during the day. I have lost tons of sleep due to many 2 am ice cream runs for my wife. At least I got to eat some ice cream, too!

- **Morning sickness is just for mornings.**

Yet another myth! While morning sickness could be called that for a reason, it is not exclusively a morning thing. A pregnant woman can feel nauseous or unwell for several reasons due to certain smells, tastes of foods and drinks, and other things. Light nausea is perfectly normal. But it can happen throughout the day, not just in the morning. Ginger candies and aromatherapy really helped my wife get through the nausea of pregnancy. If your partner's nausea is severe to the point where she cannot eat, you should consider contacting your healthcare provider for tips.

So we've seen some of the most common myths related to pregnancy. You and your partner might be showered with these during the expecting period, but don't take them all to heart. Despite how convincing some pregnancy myths may sound, they are called myths for a reason: they lack scientific evidence and often stem from simple cultural beliefs or outdated information. These myths can spread quickly through word of mouth, social media, or even well-intentioned but misinformed family and friends. While they may seem plausible or even logical, it is crucial to approach them with skepticism and seek evidence-based information.

After all, the world of pregnancy is a fertile ground for such myths to take root. From old wives' tales to urban legends, these myths can cover various topics, including diet and nutrition, exercise, baby's sex prediction, labor and delivery, and postpartum care. Some myths may focus on the supposed impact of specific foods or activities on the baby's development. In contrast, others may offer shortcuts or miraculous remedies to ease common pregnancy discomforts.

However, it is essential to remember that pregnancy is a complex biological process, and decisions regarding health and well-being should be based on accurate information backed by scientific research. Many myths arise from a lack of understanding about how the human body works during pregnancy, leading to misconceptions that can potentially harm both your partner and your developing child. By examining these myths critically and consulting trusted healthcare professionals, women can gain a deeper understanding of their bodies and make informed choices throughout their pregnancy journey.

Relying on evidence-based knowledge allows expectant parents to distinguish between fact and fiction, ensuring the well-being of themselves and their babies.

Of course, it is also noteworthy to understand that your experience and your partner's experiences are unique. Pregnancy is a distinctive and individual experience that can vary significantly from person to person. Numerous factors contribute to this individuality, shaping the course and outcomes of pregnancy. The *National Institute of Child Health and Human Development (NICHD)* provides valuable insights into these factors that make pregnancy different for each person. Let's explore some of them:

- **Maternal age**: The age at which a person becomes pregnant can influence the pregnancy experience. Women younger than 20 or older than 35 may face specific challenges and potential risks. For instance, teenage pregnancies have an increased risk of preterm birth. In contrast, advanced maternal age is associated with a higher likelihood of chromosomal abnormalities.
- **Overall health**: Your partner's general health before and during pregnancy plays a significant role in pregnancy outcomes. Pre-existing medical conditions such as diabetes, hypertension, obesity, or autoimmune disorders can affect her and your developing baby. Maintaining good overall health through regular check-ups, a balanced diet, exercise, and necessary medical management is vital.

- **Genetic factors**: Genetic factors can influence various aspects of pregnancy. Inherited conditions, family history of genetic disorders, and certain genetic traits can impact the health of both the mother and the baby. Genetic counseling and prenatal testing can help identify potential risks and guide decision-making.
- **Reproductive history**: Previous experiences with pregnancy, such as prior pregnancies, miscarriages, stillbirths, or complications, can influence subsequent pregnancies. For example, women with a history of preterm birth may require additional monitoring and care during subsequent pregnancies.
- **Lifestyle factors**: Individual lifestyle choices, such as smoking, alcohol or substance abuse, and poor nutrition, can significantly affect pregnancy. These factors can increase the risk of complications, developmental issues, and long-term health problems for both the mother and the baby. A healthy lifestyle with proper nutrition, avoiding harmful substances, and maintaining physical and mental well-being, is essential for a successful and healthy pregnancy.
- **Socioeconomic factors**: Socioeconomic status can impact the accessibility and quality of prenatal care, nutrition, and support systems available to pregnant individuals. Financial stability, education, and social support networks can influence the pregnancy experience and outcomes.

Recognizing that each person's pregnancy journey is unique and influenced by a combination of these factors is crucial.

Healthcare providers consider these individual factors when providing personalized care and support throughout pregnancy. By understanding these factors and working closely with healthcare professionals, you and your partner can navigate the pregnancy journey with excellent knowledge and confidence, ensuring the best possible outcomes for you and your baby.

Of course, this is not an invitation for you to make your own conclusions and take things lightly. Pregnancy is one of the most critical stages of your life and your relationship and must be taken seriously. That is why you must consult your doctor before doing anything you need clarification on. Your obstetrician - the physician specializing in delivering babies and caring for people during pregnancy and after birth - should be your leading source of all pregnancy-related information. It is always best to direct your questions to them, knowing that the answers will have credibility and be tailored precisely for you.

THE EXPECTANT FATHER'S SIDE OF PREGNANCY

Pregnancy is a transformative experience and the journey of a lifetime - but not just for the birthing partner. You, the non-birthing partner, may not experience the same physical and emotional changes your partner does. However, you still play a crucial role in supporting and navigating pregnancy's emotional and practical aspects. Moreover, there is some evidence that expectant fathers may also experience hormone changes! Nature has its own secret ways, and it orchestrates everything according to the grand plan of *life*. So, to become the best possible partner and father, you too may experience some "behind the scenes" changes.

On the basic level, these changes might be physical. If you begin noticing a bit of added weight and slight curves on your belly, there could be a reason for that! Studies show that men may gain a few extra pounds when expecting a child. This is nature's way of ensuring that - when the time comes - you will be in good condition to care for and provide for the child and the mother.

Another reason for such changes is because of hormones. That's right; fluctuating hormone levels are not experienced only by mothers - men can experience them too. When they become parents - or are about to - men's testosterone levels will fall. The most significant male hormone, testosterone, is impor-tant when you are young and in your prime - it serves as the driving force in your search for a partner. But when your mission is accomplished, and a baby is on the way, your testos-terone levels can drop as the focus shifts towards building strong relationships and caring for your baby.

Of course, the changes you experience during pregnancy can be complex and multi-dimensional, affecting your character. During these transformative nine months, you will see your partner changing physically and emotionally. As her body conditions for the all-important role of motherhood, women will change in many ways. You, the non-birthing partner, will have to adopt the function of a protector and supporter and master the skills of empathy, understanding, and patience. The two of you form the nucleus of your emerging family. You must create a safe space for open communication, ensuring that every critical moment passes with mutual support and understanding. Just remember that expectant fathers play a significant role in providing emotional and physical support throughout the entire journey. This may involve offering a listening ear, being understanding during challenging moments, providing comfort measures for physical discomfort, and assisting with household chores or other practical tasks as your partner's energy levels fluctuate. Now is the time to be the rock of the relationship by standing firm in the face of any new challenges during these nine months and beyond.

Likewise, pregnancy may require certain lifestyle adjustments for you as the expectant father. This could involve supporting the pregnant person in adopting a healthy diet by helping prepare food, encouraging regular exercise, and creating a nurturing and safe environment at home. It may also mean changing daily routines and activities to accommodate your partner's needs and comfort.

These things will be challenging. Sometimes, you can't be in your prime and be one hundred percent supportive. In these cases, stress can accumulate, and things will become overwhelming. That is why it is vital to find a way to let loose that slow build-up of pressure and get back in the groove as quickly as you can. Find time during the day for a hobby or relaxing activity, solo or with your partner. Even if it's something quick, it can be satisfying and allow you to replenish your energy. My stress relief came through playing a short video game, doing a quick workout, or taking a short nap.

Most importantly, however, you might experience new moments and changes in the relationship with your partner. It's no secret that pregnancy can sometimes put pressure on your relationship and lead to arguments and miscommunication. Depending on the circumstances, you might also be influenced by worry. Fears about money, your partner's well-being, or specific limitations are common. They should not dictate your everyday mood or your personal relationships. Other factors that can strain your connection are the lack of sex and intimacy.

After all, in certain stages of the pregnancy journey, you both may feel differently about having sex or being passionate about it. Open and honest communication and understanding become vital as both partners navigate impending parenthood's new roles and responsibilities. With good conversation, an open mind, and knowledge, you can quickly bridge the differences and look at the situation from a fresh and normal angle.

Remember that you and your partner are working together - you are a team on a path to victory. And as long as you remain open, honest, and supportive, that path will be straight and smooth.

YOUR PARTNER'S PREGNANCY AND YOUR EMOTIONS

It's time to talk - *man to man* - and face some straightforward facts. Now that we've taken a plunge into this pregnancy survival guide, some things are beginning to settle. You are on a journey toward fatherhood, and that's no small thing. In many ways, you are opening a new chapter of your life that will leave you happy, fulfilled, and more mature. And I understand if that sounds like a paramount thing at times - because it is. Feeling a range of conflicting emotions, entirely new feelings, and feeling overwhelmed are completely normal things that you shouldn't shy away from. They are all a part of a man's journey through life - and will definitely leave you stronger and more complete as an individual.

It is typical for expectant fathers to experience a wide range of emotions, feelings, and fears during pregnancy. Being an expecting father is monumental, after all!

- **Fear:** Throughout this journey, you might feel fear - especially that pesky *fear of the unknown.* First-time fathers are especially hounded by many worries. After all, they have embarked upon a journey whose first and foremost stage begins in nine months. Concerns about the health and well-being of your partner and your baby, financial pressures, changes in the relationship dynamic, and the challenges of becoming a parent can evoke anxiety and worry. Sometimes, such feelings are not to be avoided. Instead, you should embrace them and understand that they are a passing thing and that - in the end - everything will be just as it should be.
- **New Roles:** The pregnancy journey creates a new set of roles for you as a first-time dad. You could face unique challenges daily, and your well-established routine could "take a beating." Because of this, it is necessary to adapt. Try and adjust your daily schedule to meet new

responsibilities and tasks. Also, it is important to always find time for your partner, as she will require your presence and support in pregnancy-related matters. Although it won't be easy, it may be time to make changes to meet her needs.

- **Helplessness and Confusion:** Expectant fathers may also grapple with their own response to the physical and emotional changes their partner is experiencing. Witnessing the physical discomforts, hormonal shifts, and mood swings can evoke feelings of helplessness or confusion. Remember that pregnancy can be an emotionally demanding time for your partner, and having a stable and supportive father-to-be can significantly impact their well-being. By managing your emotions, you can provide a calming presence and offer the necessary emotional support throughout the pregnancy journey.

YOU CAN A.C.E. THIS!

The A.C.E. method (Awareness, Connection, Embrace) can help you look at pregnancy and fatherhood in a totally new light. Expectant fathers are crucial for a positive pregnancy experience. Still, many dads must know their significance and role in perinatal care. Traditionally, the role of fathers during pregnancy and childbirth has been somewhat overshadowed by the spotlight being set on the expectant mother's experience. Throughout history, fathers were often excluded from the birthing process. They were expected to provide financial support and protection rather than emotional or physical care.

These deeply ingrained societal norms and expectations have contributed to a lack of awareness among fathers regarding their role in perinatal care.

Luckily, over the years, there has been a shift in societal attitudes, recognizing the importance of fathers' involvement in pregnancy and childbirth. Research has highlighted the positive impact of paternal engagement on maternal and infant outcomes. However, disseminating this knowledge to fathers and promoting their active participation in perinatal care remains challenging despite these advancements. That is why, as the first step of the A.C.E. method, you must raise your awareness. It's time that we dispel those aged preconceptions entirely and improve the beliefs and knowledge of men. *You* matter. *You* are needed. Without *you*, your partner can't thrive as they should, especially in this critical and challenging period of their life.

Awareness:

To successfully raise your awareness about all things pregnancy and fatherhood related, it is essential to educate yourself. Luckily, you are already tackling that first step while reviewing these pages. You would be surprised at how much pregnancy, birth, and aftercare improve when fathers become educated and prepared for the entire process. Fathers can educate themselves through books and online resources, attending prenatal classes, and engaging in open and honest conversations with their partners. By understanding the various stages of pregnancy and the challenges that may arise, fathers can better empathize with their partners and provide appropriate support. Awareness of one's role, being proactive in learning about the implications of pregnancy on overall well-being, and connecting with others, including their partners, can significantly contribute to a father's sense of security and confidence.

Connection:

It is so vital to connect - not only with your partner but also with others. Expectant fathers must establish a solid emotional connection with their partners during pregnancy. Open communication, active participation in prenatal appointments, and expressing support and empathy can foster a deeper bond. Engaging in shared activities like reading pregnancy-related books together, attending birthing classes, and discussing birth plans can further strengthen the connection. By actively involving themselves in the pregnancy journey, fathers demonstrate their commitment and support, which helps their partners feel secure and valued. But it is critical to connect with those around you as well. Engaging with other fathers, support groups, and communities can provide invaluable support and insights. Connecting with individuals with similar experiences or challenges allows fathers to share their concerns, exchange advice, and learn from one another. This networking creates a sense of belonging, normalizes their experiences, and provides a platform to discuss topics related to fatherhood and pregnancy openly. Such connections can boost fathers' confidence and offer practical tips for navigating the journey.

Embrace:

The final element of the A.C.E. method is embracing the transformative nature of pregnancy and embracing the new roles and responsibilities that come with fatherhood. This includes actively supporting the mother in physical and emotional aspects. Fathers can contribute by assisting with household chores, accompanying their partners on errands, preparing nutritious meals, and encouraging self-care. Additionally, fathers should be ready for the emotional ups and downs that may occur during pregnancy and be available to provide a listening ear, understanding, and reassurance. Embrace your supportive role! It's time to be that foundation of support and reliance!

So, we've tackled those key first steps and tips that every dad-to-be needs to hear and take in, from understanding your new position to accepting the changes that it inevitably brings, all the way to raising your awareness, connecting with your part-ner, and embracing this incredible new journey that the two of you are embarking on. In the following chapters, we will discuss what you should expect during every crucial step of each trimester of pregnancy.

2

THE FIRST TRIMESTER

I t's time to get in the groove. Remember, you're here for a reason and are *very* special. Why? Because the miracle of life is, in fact, very, very special. The odds of being alive and born are remarkable when considering the many factors that had to align perfectly throughout time and history. The universe is vast and predominantly inhospitable to life as we know it. Countless factors had to align for our planet, Earth, to possess the right conditions for life to emerge and thrive. Life on Earth has gone through billions of years of evolution, leading to the diverse species we see today. This process of evolution requires an intricate interplay between genetic mutations, natural selection, and adaptation to changing environments. The odds of any specific organism evolving and surviving to the point of reproducing and passing on its genes are incredibly slim.

Tracing our ancestral lineage reveals an unbroken chain of successful reproduction that stretches back thousands of years. Every one of our ancestors faced countless challenges and survived long enough to reproduce, ensuring that their genetic material would be passed down through the generations. On an individual level, the odds of a specific person being conceived and born are astronomically low. Consider the millions of sperm competing to fertilize an egg during conception. The specific combination of one particular sperm and one specific egg had to occur out of countless possibilities for each person to come into existence. And, with all that being said - here *you* are now. Against incredible odds, life won - and you, a unique and special person, are here now, reading this book. How amazing is that? Even more remarkable is that you and your partner are now nurturing another life whose presence in this world will be another triumph against incredible odds.

That said, it is necessary to remember that conceiving a child is sometimes more effortful than it may seem. While some individuals may become pregnant quickly and easily, it can be challenging and emotionally taxing for others. Whatever the case was for you and your partner, you've done it! You continued that unbroken lineage that stretches back thousands of years. And that's a *big* thing.

In those first few weeks of your pregnancy journey, things could still seem as they were before you found out the big news. There are no visible changes, your daily routine is still the same, and the only thing you have left is knowing that a tiny fetus grows steadily with each new day. But things will change, and soon at that. It might not seem like it, but during weeks 1 and 2 of pregnancy, significant changes occur in a woman's body, even though conception and implantation of the fertilized egg typically happen during week 2. It's important to note that pregnancy is commonly measured from the first day of the woman's last menstrual period (L.M.P.), so the actual conception occurs around two weeks later.

Let's discuss what happens in the early stages. There is a lot of medical terminology to run through, but I'll try to make it as simple and painless as possible.

Weeks 1 and 2: Menstruation and Ovulation

In the first week of pregnancy, a woman is typically menstruating (bleeding) as the uterine lining sheds in response to the absence of a fertilized egg. However, this bleeding is not related to pregnancy but rather the beginning of a new menstrual cycle. In a typical 28-day menstrual cycle, ovulation usually occurs around day 14. The ovary releases an egg into the fallopian tube, where it awaits meeting the sperm.

Week 3: Conception

Week 3 marks the beginning of pregnancy as conception occurs during this period.

Conception: When sexual intercourse occurs around ovulation, sperm can travel through the cervix, uterus, and into the fallopian tube to meet the egg. Fertilization happens when one sperm successfully penetrates and merges with the egg, forming a single cell called a zygote.

- Cell Division and Migration: After fertilization, the zygote begins a process of rapid cell division, forming a cluster of cells called a blastocyst. Over the next few days, the blastocyst migrates down the fallopian tube toward the uterus.

Week 4: Implantation, Transformation, and Organogenesis

By Week 4, the blastocyst reaches the uterus and seeks a suitable spot for implantation. It burrows into the uterine lining and connects with the mother's circulatory system through specialized structures known as the placenta and umbilical cord. These connections allow the exchange of nutrients and waste between the mother and the developing embryo. During weeks 1 and 2, a woman may not be aware that she is pregnant since it is still very early. It usually takes a few more weeks before pregnancy symptoms, such as missed periods or hormonal changes, become noticeable. At this stage, taking care of one's health, such as avoiding alcohol and tobacco, maintaining a balanced diet, and taking prenatal vitamins if trying to conceive, can contribute to the overall well-being of the developing embryo. During weeks 3 and 4 of pregnancy, significant developments occur as the fertilized egg grows and implants further into the uterine lining. The embryo begins to form, and essential structures and systems start to take shape.

The fertilized egg is still a cluster of cells (blastocyte). However, by the end of the week, it transforms into an embryo, marking the start of significant developmental changes.

The placenta begins to develop, and blood vessels form to establish a connection between the mother and the growing embryo.

Another critical element, the neural tube, which will later develop into the brain and spinal cord, begins to take shape. This is a crucial phase, and proper nutrition, including sufficient folic acid intake, is vital for preventing neural tube defects.

Week 4 also marks the beginning of organogenesis, a phase where the basic structures of major organs and systems start to form. The heart starts to develop and beat, initially as a simple tube. Blood vessels begin to assemble, and the circulatory system takes shape. The primitive structures of other vital organs, such as the brain, spinal cord, lungs, liver, and kidneys, begin to develop. Although they are still in their early stages, their formation sets the foundation for further growth and specialization.

- Amniotic Sac and Umbilical Cord: The amniotic sac, filled with amniotic fluid, envelops and protects the developing embryo. The umbilical cord, which connects the embryo to the placenta, starts to form and provides the embryo with essential nutrients and oxygen.
- Confirmation of Pregnancy: Towards the end of week 4, a woman may notice some early signs of pregnancy, such as a missed period, breast tenderness, fatigue, or mild nausea. These symptoms are often the first indications that a pregnancy has occurred. So, as you

see, pregnancy starts to take shape during its fourth week, and many couples only realize it then.

These developmental milestones are general guidelines and can vary from person to person. Expectant mothers should maintain a healthy lifestyle, including a balanced diet, regular exercise, prenatal care, and avoiding substances harmful to the developing embryo, such as alcohol and tobacco. Consulting with healthcare professionals throughout the pregnancy journey is essential to ensure the well-being of both your partner and the growing embryo.

So, as we see, during these first four weeks of pregnancy, fetal development is focused on the very early stages of conception and implantation. The baby - i.e., the fetus - is in its simplest form and will only subsequently begin taking a more "natural" shape.

THE SECOND MONTH

It's important to note that the organs and structures are forming during these early stages, as many critical developments occur. As mentioned, exposure to harmful substances or certain medications during this time can affect the embryo's normal development.

And with that, you and your partner are now entirely in the pregnancy journey. It is a fantastic feeling, as you will realize, knowing that a little bundle of life is forming within your partner. Over the next nine months, you both will experience many new things and see many changes. Yet, you will notice few *visible* physical changes in these first four weeks. But what about the second month? What happens in weeks 5 and 6? During this time, the embryo continues to change rapidly, and several significant changes occur. Here's an overview of the key developments during this period:

Week 5:

- The embryo is now about 3-4 mm long, roughly the size of a sesame seed.
- The brain and spinal cord begin to take shape, and the neural tube, which will become the brain and spinal cord, closes completely.
- The heart continues to develop and beats at a regular rhythm. Ultrasound may detect it around the end of week 5 or the beginning of week 6.
- The circulatory system starts to form with the early development of blood vessels.
- Facial features, such as eyes, ears, and nostrils, begin to appear as small indentations.
- Bud-like structures form for the arms and legs, eventually growing and developing into limbs.
- The digestive system starts to develop, including the formation of the esophagus, stomach, and intestines.

Week 6:

- The embryo grows to approximately 5-6 mm in length.

- The head becomes more prominent, and facial features continue to develop, including the formation of the mouth and tongue.
- Small indentations appear where the future eyes and ears will be located.
- The limb buds become more defined and show signs of early hand and foot development.
- The respiratory system starts to form, with the formation of the trachea and lung buds.
- The heart continues to grow and develop, and blood circulation becomes more efficient.
- The placenta continues to develop and take over the role of providing oxygen and nutrients to the growing embryo.
- The umbilical cord, which connects the embryo to the placenta, becomes more distinct and contains blood vessels facilitating nutrient exchange.
- During weeks 5-6, although the embryo is still tiny, it undergoes significant transformations as major organs and systems begin to develop.

Of course, changes are reserved not only for the developing embryo but also for the mother. As her body adapts to the early stages of pregnancy, a woman may experience various physical and emotional changes. Here are some of the most common changes that may occur in your partner during weeks 5 and 6:

- Her breasts may become tender, swollen, or sensitive. Her nipples may darken, and the veins in the breast area may become more prominent.

- Increased levels of progesterone can cause feelings of fatigue and exhaustion. Your partner's body is working hard to support the developing embryo.
- Some women may start experiencing morning sickness, including nausea, vomiting, or food aversions. It's important to note that not all women experience morning sickness, and it can vary in severity.
- The growing uterus puts pressure on the bladder, leading to more frequent urination.
- Hormonal changes can lead to mood swings, irritability, or emotional ups and downs.
- Some women may develop specific cravings for certain foods. In contrast, others may experience aversions to smells or tastes they previously enjoyed.
- It's common for her to have a slightly increased vaginal discharge during pregnancy. However, if there is a significant change in color, odor, or consistency, please consult a healthcare provider for recommendations.
- Hormonal changes can affect digestion, leading to bloating, gas, and constipation.
- Some women may notice that their sense of smell becomes more sensitive during pregnancy, which can contribute to food aversions or nausea.

Within the first trimester, the embryo develops quite rapidly. That is just another miracle of life! During weeks 7 and 8, the embryo undergoes significant changes as it transforms into a recognizable human form. First, ultrasounds around this time can show a recognizable outline of a human embryo. However, it's important to note that the embryo is still in the early stages of development, and the organs and systems continue to mature. Here are some of the changes that occur around this time:

Week 7:

- The embryo is now approximately 10-12 mm long, roughly the size of a blueberry.
- Facial features become more distinct. The eyes, which initially developed as indentations, are now more prominent and have eyelid folds forming. The nose, mouth, and ears continue to grow.
- The brain continues to expand with the formation of different regions.
- The arm and legs grow longer and become more defined, with webbed fingers and toes forming.
- The embryonic tail, which was present earlier, starts to disappear.
- The heart continues to develop and beat at a faster rate.
- The major organs and systems, such as the lungs, liver, kidneys, and digestive systems, continue developing.
- The umbilical cord, connecting the embryo to the placenta, grows longer and becomes more complex.
- The sex organs begin to differentiate, although it may not be possible to determine the baby's sex through ultrasound yet.

Week 8:

- The embryo is now approximately 16-18 mm long, about the size of a kidney bean.
- The facial features become more refined, with the eyes moving closer together and the eyelids covering the developing eyes.
- The nose starts to take shape, and the mouth develops tooth buds.
- The external ears become more noticeable.
- The arms and legs continue to grow longer and show the beginnings of fingers and toes.
- The brain continues to develop rapidly, and the head constitutes a larger portion of the body.
- The digestive system continues to develop, with the formation of the intestines.
- The heart is divided into four chambers and is fully formed.
- The placenta continues growing and supplying the embryo with oxygen and nutrients.
- The amniotic sac, which surrounds the developing fetus, is filled with amniotic fluid that provides protection and cushioning.

THE THIRD MONTH

Time flies! You and your partner are already entering the third month of your pregnancy journey. At this point in time, you may or may not see an itty bitty "baby bump." A prominent stomach may occur only in the third trimester for some women. Everyone's built differently, so don't worry if your partner still isn't "showing ."

What is more, in the third month, the embryo enters the *fetus* stage. The basic structures and systems are in place, and the fetus exhibits more human-like features. The coming weeks will bring further development and maturation of organs and the growth of body proportions. Regular prenatal care, including check-ups and screenings, becomes increasingly important during this stage of pregnancy. It is crucial to contact your appointed doctor, who will schedule appointments regularly. Here are some of the pivotal developments that will occur during the third month:

Week 9:

- The embryo is now referred to as a fetus. It measures approximately 2.5-3 centimeters in length, similar to the size of a grape.
- Facial features become more refined. The eyes move closer together, and the eyelids fuse shut to protect the developing eyes.
- The external ears are well-formed.
- The head is still large compared to the rest of the body, but it becomes more proportional.
- The limbs continue to grow and develop, with the fingers and toes becoming distinct and separating from the webbing.
- Muscles, bones, and joints develop further, enabling movement and reflexes.
- The reproductive organs continue to develop, but it may still be challenging to determine the baby's sex through ultrasound.

- The liver produces red blood cells until the bone marrow takes over this function later in pregnancy.
- The diaphragm, which is crucial for breathing, develops.

Week 10:

- The fetus grows to about 3.8-5.1 centimeters in length, approximately the size of a strawberry.
- Facial features continue to develop, including the formation of the nose, nostrils, and lips.
- The head remains prominent, but the facial profile becomes more distinct.
- The eyes, initially on the sides of the head, move closer together, and the eyelids remain fused.
- The tiny tooth buds form within the gums.
- The fingers and toes are fully separated, and the nails begin to develop.
- The skeleton, previously cartilaginous, starts to harden into bone.
- The fetus makes spontaneous movements, although your partner has not yet felt them.
- The placenta continues to grow and provide nourishment and oxygen to the developing fetus.
- The amniotic fluid increases, providing protection and cushioning.

Week 11:

- The fetus now measures around 5.1-6.4 centimeters long, about the size of a lime.
- Facial features continue to develop and become more refined. The eyes are fully formed, and the eyelids remain closed.
- The ears are positioned correctly on the sides of the head.
- The neck becomes more defined, allowing for better movement.
- The external genitals may start to show differentiation. However, it can still be challenging to determine the baby's sex through ultrasound.
- The limbs continue to grow and develop, with muscles becoming prominent.
- Nails begin to form on the fingers and toes.
- The digestive system matures further, and the intestines move from the umbilical cord into the abdominal cavity.
- The pancreas starts producing insulin.
- The fetus begins to make swallowing movements and can urinate small amounts of urine.
- The fetus becomes more active, although the mother may not feel these movements yet.

Week 12:

- The fetus grows to around 6.4-7.6 centimeters in length, similar to the size of a plum.
- The facial features become more distinct, with the upper lip and palate forming.
- The eyes are still fused shut.
- The scalp hair begins to develop.
- The bones continue to harden, and the skeletal structure becomes more defined.
- Swallowing and sucking reflexes become more coordinated.
- The placenta provides all the necessary nutrients and oxygen, eliminating waste products through the umbilical cord.
- The kidneys produce urine.
- The liver starts making bile.
- The vocal cords begin to form.
- The uterus expands to accommodate the growing fetus, causing the mother's abdomen to become more rounded.

Three months already passed - just six more to go! In the above segment, we took a detailed glimpse into the intricate developments of your baby. Even though the fetus is relatively small at this point, you can see its recognizable outlines on your appointed ultrasound. It is a feeling quite unlike any other - so cherish the moment. You will be surprised at how time can slip away, and before you know it, that tiny little blob on the medical screen will be a happy and loved little baby.

The first trimester, however, is critical as a formative stage where the foundations for healthy further development are laid down. So, as a caring and responsible partner, you should ensure that your pregnant partner enjoys all the benefits and comforts - as much as possible. The first stages of pregnancy are experienced differently in certain parts of the world. Many pregnant women remain in their workplace for the first few months of pregnancy and even up to 9 months in some parts of the world. Of course, in the ideal society, your partner should rest and relax for the entire 9-month gestation period, living a healthy lifestyle that will benefit both her and the baby. Remember, these first few weeks, as the embryo takes shapes and forms into a fetus, are very delicate, so encourage your partner to ditch some old unhealthy habits (if there are any) and try adopting something new and refreshing as a change in your lifestyle. You'd be surprised at how a few small changes can benefit the entire family.

CHANGES IN YOUR PARTNER

The first trimester is also when you start noticing changes in your partner. You will observe, first-hand, how the woman you know and love changes in appearance and character. Here is a mother-to-be, delicate yet strong, changed - yet beautiful. The changes you will see are, of course, physical. Here are just a few of the things to expect:

- Her body produces higher levels of estrogen and progesterone to support pregnancy, so your partner could exhibit mood swings and different emotions and gain a few extra pounds. All of this is perfectly normal.

- Her metabolism increases, and blood volume gradually expands to accommodate the growing fetus. This can result in increased appetite and different energy levels.
- The heart works harder to pump the increased blood volume, leading to an increased heart rate. Often enough, when your partner's heart beats faster, you shouldn't be worried. Some rest and relaxation are all that's needed.
- Hormonal changes can slow digestion, leading to bloating, constipation, and heartburn. These are common occurrences in the first trimester.
- The immune system may become slightly suppressed to prevent the body from rejecting the developing fetus.

Of course, changes are not only physiological but can be emotional and psychological.

- Hormonal fluctuations can cause mood swings, irritability, and emotional changes.
- Women may experience heightened emotional sensitivity or feel more emotional overall.
- The anticipation and responsibility of becoming a parent can lead to both anxiety and excitement.

Every woman's experience during the first trimester can differ. While some may experience mild symptoms, others may face more pronounced discomfort. If any concerns arise or if the woman experiences severe symptoms, it's essential to consult a healthcare provider for guidance and support throughout the first trimester and the remainder of the pregnancy.

THE POSSIBILITY OF MISCARRIAGE

Alas, we cannot avoid mentioning one aspect of early pregnancy - miscarriage. Sadly, this is something that is always a possibility in pregnancy and the way nature works. It doesn't happen often, and you shouldn't be focused only on that aspect, worrying too much. But it is worth knowing the basics. A miscarriage is the loss of a pregnancy before 20 weeks gestation. Most miscarriages happen in the first trimester of pregnancy, typically within the first 12 weeks, so we must mention it. The exact cause of miscarriage can often be tricky to determine, but various factors can contribute to its occurrence. The most common cause of miscarriage in the first trimester is chromosomal abnormalities in the fetus. These abnormalities occur randomly during fertilization or due to errors in cell division. Moreover, chromosomal abnormalities are often incompatible with life, leading to spontaneous miscarriage as the body recognizes the anomaly and terminates the pregnancy.

Another possible cause is an imbalance in the hormones, particularly progesterone, which can impact the stability of the uterine lining and the ability to maintain a pregnancy. Insufficient levels of progesterone, a very important hormone, can cause the uterus to contract and expel the developing embryo. Other causes that can increase the risk of miscarriage are certain maternal health conditions, such as poorly controlled diabetes, thyroid disorders, or autoimmune diseases.

Infections, such as bacterial vaginosis, urinary tract infections, or sexually transmitted infections, can also contribute. Of course, it goes without saying that certain lifestyle factors can significantly increase the risk of miscarriage, including smoking, alcohol consumption, drug use, and exposure to environmental toxins. It is critical that your partner avoids alcohol, drugs, or any other toxins throughout pregnancy, especially in this early stage of pregnancy, as they can cause various types of developmental issues in the fetus if miscarriage does not occur.

Miscarriage can manifest differently for each woman, and symptoms can vary. Common signs of a miscarriage include vaginal bleeding, cramping, and the passing of tissue. However, some miscarriages may occur without noticeable symptoms, and the loss may only be detected during routine prenatal checks or ultrasound examinations. If your partner experiences symptoms suggestive of a miscarriage, it is crucial to seek immediate medical attention. Your healthcare provider will perform a physical exam, possibly including an ultrasound, to determine if a miscarriage has occurred. Sometimes, medical intervention may be necessary to complete the miscarriage and ensure the woman's health.

Looking back into history, into the times of our great-grandparents, we can quickly see that they experienced a lot of loss, as miscarriages often happened at those times. Today, however, miscarriages are not so common, but they can still occur often enough. It is essential to know the signs and symptoms of a potential miscarriage. When a miscarriage happens, it refers to the loss of a pregnancy before the 20th week. Miscarriages can occur for various reasons, often related to genetic abnormalities or problems with the development of the fetus. It's important to note that miscarriages can affect about 10-20% of known pregnancies. How do you know that something is wrong?

- **Vaginal bleeding:** This can range from light spotting to heavy bleeding. While light spotting doesn't always indicate a problem, contacting a healthcare provider is essential if bleeding is heavy or accompanied by severe pain.
- **Cramping or abdominal pain**: Mild cramping during early pregnancy can be expected, but a healthcare professional should evaluate persistent or severe abdominal pain.
- **Loss of pregnancy symptoms**: If common pregnancy symptoms, such as breast tenderness or nausea, suddenly disappear, it could be a sign of a miscarriage or other complications.
- **Tissue passing:** Passing tissue or clots from the vagina may indicate a miscarriage, especially if accompanied by bleeding and cramping
- **Signs of premature labor:** Premature labor refers to the onset of labor before the 37th week of pregnancy. It is a concerning situation that requires immediate medical attention. Signs of premature labor include:

  ○ Regular contractions that occur more than four times per hour or every 10 minutes
  ○ Increase in vaginal discharge, especially if it is watery, bloody, or mucus-like

○ Pelvic pressure or a feeling of the baby pushing down
○ Lower back pain that is constant or comes and goes
○ Abdominal cramping or menstrual-like cramps
○ Rupture of the membranes (breaking of the water)

When to call a doctor? It's important to contact a healthcare provider promptly if any of the following situations occur:

- Vaginal bleeding that is heavy or accompanied by severe pain
- Severe or persistent abdominal pain or cramping
- Noticeable decrease in fetal movement
- Leakage of fluid from the vagina
- Signs of infection include fever, chills, or unusual vaginal discharge
- Any concerns or questions regarding the pregnancy's progression or the mother's or baby's health

It is essential to provide support and understanding to women who experience a miscarriage, as it can be highly emotional and distressing. Counseling and support groups are available to help cope with the grief and emotions associated with the loss. In the case of a miscarriage or concerns about pregnancy complications, healthcare providers are the best resource for guidance, diagnosis, and appropriate medical care. They can evaluate individual symptoms, perform necessary examinations or tests, and provide support during challenging situations. Experiencing a miscarriage can be a profoundly emotional and difficult time for both partners. It is vital to support and under-stand each other during this difficult period. Here are some tips and advice on how to support a partner when going through a miscarriage:

- **Open Communication:** Encourage open and honest communication with your partner. Allow them to express their emotions, fears, and concerns without judgment. Be available to listen and offer a shoulder to lean on. Share your own feelings and experiences, as it can help create a sense of empathy and connection.
- **Validate Their Emotions:** Understand that grief and loss manifest differently for each person. Validate your partner's emotions and let them know their feelings are appropriate. Avoid minimizing or dismissing their pain. Offer reassurance that it is okay to grieve and that you are there to support them throughout the process.
- **Be Empathetic and Patient:** Recognize that the grieving process takes time and that healing occurs at different paces for different individuals. Be patient with your partner's emotional ups and downs. Offer empathy and understanding without rushing their recovery or imposing a specific timeline on their grief.
- **Provide Physical and Practical Support:** Attend medical appointments together, accompany your partner during procedures, and provide physical comfort. Offer assistance with household chores, errands, and tasks that may feel overwhelming during this time. Small gestures of kindness and support can make a significant difference.
- **Seek Counseling or Support Groups:** Consider attending counseling sessions or seeking support from

support groups specifically tailored to individuals and couples who have experienced pregnancy loss. Professional guidance and connecting with others who have gone through similar experiences can provide additional avenues for healing and coping.

- **Take Care of Yourself:** Taking care of yourself during this challenging time is equally important. Ensure you have your own support system, seek counseling if needed, and practice self-care to manage your own emotions and well-being. You will be better equipped to support your partner by remembering to care for yourself.

The impacts of a miscarriage can be profound for both partners. Emotionally, individuals may experience grief, sadness, guilt, anger, and a sense of loss. It can strain the couple's relationship and lead to feelings of isolation or failure. Supporting each other is necessary for navigating these challenges together. When enough time passes, a couple can try again - life and love always find a way to triumph.

HOW TO A.C.E. THE FIRST TRIMESTER!

Awareness:

During the first trimester, you must realize that prenatal care is crucial. You can choose from an obstetrician, a midwife, group prenatal care, or a family physician. All options are viable, but taking care of those first few prenatal appointments is mandatory. Prenatal care is critically important for the health and well-being of the pregnant woman and the developing fetus. The first appointment should be made when you confirm that you and your partner are expecting. These visits allow monitoring of the mother's health, including blood pressure, weight, and overall well-being. Potential health issues or complications can be identified and addressed early, reducing the risk of adverse outcomes. Prenatal care includes various screenings and tests to assess the growth and development of the fetus. Ultrasounds, blood tests, and other diagnostic procedures can detect potential fetal abnormalities or risks.

Moreover, prenatal care allows expectant parents to receive education, counseling, and emotional support. Topics covered may include childbirth preparation, breastfeeding, newborn care, and postpartum well-being. This support helps parents feel more confident, informed, and prepared for pregnancy, childbirth, and parenthood.

On your first visit, you can expect your doctor to inquire about your partner's last menstrual cycle, a family medical history, any medications you take, your lifestyle, and similar things. Providing accurate information is crucial so the doctor can take the best care of you and your baby. Share information about sensitive issues like domestic abuse or past drug use. Anything that can help paint a clear and detailed picture of your partner's health and pregnancy will be necessary.

Of course, you will learn your "due date" on your prenatal appointment. This is the time at which your partner will be 40 weeks pregnant. Please remember that this is the estimated due date, not your child's birth date. This simple "guideline" is esti-mated based on your partner's last menstrual cycle. The esti-mated delivery date allows your chosen doctor to monitor the baby's growth and the overall progress of your pregnancy. Your due date also helps schedule tests and procedures so they are done precisely at the right time. It also gives you an overall idea when you are about to welcome your baby into the world. However, remember that babies can be born before or after the full term.

As eager and expecting parents-to-be, you naturally want to know that everything will be a-OK with your little baby. Nature, however, works in mysterious ways, and babies can come into this world with many issues and genetic defects. To make sure that your baby is developing healthily, you can do a test for fetal concerns. These tests, also known as prenatal screening and diagnostic tests, are medical procedures performed during pregnancy to assess the health and develop-ment of the fetus. These tests can provide valuable information about potential genetic disorders, chromosomal abnormalities, and other fetal conditions. The choice to undergo these tests is typically a personal decision made by the expectant parents, considering their medical history, age, and potential risk factors. One of the most common - and safest - prenatal screening methods is the so-called NIPT. This blood test analyzes fetal D.N.A. present in the mother's blood. It screens for chromosomal abnormalities, such as Down syndrome (tri-somy 21), Edwards syndrome (trisomy 18), and Patau syndrome (trisomy 13). NIPT is highly accurate and can be done as early as ten weeks into pregnancy. Still, it is considered a screening test and may require confirmatory testing for a definitive diagnosis. This test could be a bit expensive - depending on the part of the world you're from - but it goes a long way to ensure that everything is coming along smoothly. Knowing that your baby is healthy will give you peace of mind.

Connection:

One of the ideal ways to ace this ground-laying period of your pregnancy is by going to antenatal classes. An antenatal or prenatal childbirth education class is a program designed to prepare expectant parents for pregnancy, childbirth, and early parenthood. These classes are typically offered by healthcare providers, hospitals, or private organizations. They are conducted by trained instructors, such as midwives, nurses, or childbirth educators. These classes cover a wide range of crucial topics to understand and master. They provide vital education and knowledge, prepare you for childbirth, encourage the involvement of both partners, create a supportive environment, and tell you about the postpartum period. Attending antenatal care, engaging with a chosen healthcare provider, participating in antenatal classes, and connecting with other couples can significantly enhance an expectant parent's understanding of the first trimester and equip them to support their partner effectively.

Support your partner with daily activities. If your partner usually does the groceries by herself, now is your chance to accompany her and help her choose foods that will keep her and your developing baby well-nourished. If she does all the cooking, start assisting her in the kitchen, as you may have to take over as head chef in the later stages of pregnancy, depending on her energy levels and discomfort with her growing belly.

Embrace:

Attending antenatal care visits, communicating with a chosen healthcare provider, participating in antenatal classes, and connecting with other couples help you and your partner, as expectant parents, thoroughly prepare for the first trimester. It allows you to learn about pregnancy-related changes, receive medical guidance, understand the importance of prenatal care, and discover strategies to support your partner physically, emotionally, and practically during this transformative period. Take this time to embrace the changes happening in your partner as well adjustments you need to make to support her as much as possible.

And with that, we come to the close of the second chapter. The first trimester is quite important. It is the first major milestone on your pregnancy journey, a foundation towards a healthy and happy full term. New changes appear in your life, and you quickly learn to adapt and understand them. You discover how you mature with every new day, exploring the wonders of life and the joys it can bring. And as the first trimester ends, you and your partner already feel stronger and more confident about everything that will come. To that end, what comes in the second trimester?

3

THE SECOND TRIMESTER

The first three months of your new journey are already behind you. You learned some things, understood your new-found state, and recuperated from those first few shaky steps. Things seem smoother now, don't they? With each new day, there is something new, different, and certainly exciting. The important thing is this you are adapting to all the changes.

SEX DURING PREGNANCY

At this point in time, it shouldn't be all that surprising to think about… you know… being intimate. Sex is a natural thing, and sexuality is one of the fundamental cornerstones of a successful and rewarding relationship. However, during pregnancy, sex and intimacy become somewhat of a taboo subject. Without fundamental knowledge, some couples may think that sex - in any shape or form - is entirely out of the picture for nine months. But is it?

It most certainly is not. Sex is perfectly safe in pregnancy and will not harm the baby at any stage. This is provided that yours is a typical, uncomplicated pregnancy. Your baby is protected by strong uterus muscles, a mucus plug, and amniotic fluid. Having intercourse - like you always do - is completely normal. The only changes you might experience will be physical. After all, there is a baby bump in the way.

Maintaining intimacy during the second trimester of pregnancy can be an excellent way for couples to stay connected and strengthen their bond. While physical changes and discomfort may present challenges, many ways exist to enjoy a fulfilling intimate relationship. For many couples, the second trimester is when they become intimate again. This period of pregnancy is often considered a more comfortable time for many women, as the initial discomforts of the first trimester tend to subside. This can allow couples to enjoy intimacy and maintain a strong connection.

Still, don't be surprised if things don't work out as you imagined them - or with the same passion and drive as before. Your partner is pregnant, after all, and both of you can experience hormonal changes. Sex won't always be a priority on your list of activities. During pregnancy, a woman's sex drive can undergo various changes due to hormonal fluctuations, physical discomfort, and emotional factors. You are there to respect these changes and understand when it's the right time for intimacy - and when it is not.

Even if sex is not on the menu, you and your partner can still be intimate. Intimacy isn't solely about sexual activity. Embrace non-sexual forms of intimacy, such as cuddling, kissing, massages, and sharing quality time together. These activities can strengthen emotional connection and create a sense of closeness.

And sex itself has many facets. If classic penetrative sex is not comfortable, try something else! Perhaps the pregnancy will help you discover new aspects of your sexuality. Remember, every pregnancy is unique, and what works for one couple may not work for another. The key is to stay connected, communicate openly, and prioritize each other's comfort and well-being throughout the process. Sex and intimacy are, somewhat understandably, a common question topic during pregnancy. That's why it was essential to get that out of the way and put everyone's mind at ease.

ANNOUNCING THE PREGNANCY

Other critical milestones occur around this time. One of them is the announcement of your pregnancy! Announcing a pregnancy is unique from couple to couple. Some do it as soon as they find out, but many others wait for a good time when everything is certain and "set in stone." This is an exciting moment when you share your happiest news with those closest to you - those you hold dear and cherish. You can announce your pregnancy in many ways, depending on your preferences. Some only share the news with their family and friends, while others want to share it with the world.

Many couples choose to announce their pregnancy on social media platforms as well. This can be a modern and innovative approach to sharing your joy with others. You can get creative by posting a photo of an ultrasound, baby shoes, or a clever sign that hints at the upcoming arrival. Craft a heartfelt caption to accompany the image, expressing your joy and anticipation. Organize a creative photo shoot with your partner or enlist the help of a professional photographer. You can incorporate props like baby onesies, ultrasound images, or a chalkboard sign with the due date or a cute message. You or your partner can share the photos with family and friends or post them on social media.

Whatever method you choose, announcing your pregnancy will remain a personal and significant milestone in your shared journey. Staying on the same page with your partner about this is essential. There are pros and cons to waiting too long to announce your pregnancy. Wait too long, and you risk getting intrusive comments and questions regarding your partner's growing baby bump. Announce it too early, and you risk all the explaining in case the pregnancy does not succeed. Finding the balance and the right moment is key, and that will depend on you and your partner's values.

Around this stage, you are slowly approaching the midpoint of the pregnancy. This is an exciting time, and you reached it surprisingly quickly! It is also a time of new changes for your partner and baby. Here are some of the critical developments that occur during this time:

- **Quickening**: Many women start feeling their baby's first movements during the fourth month. This sensation, called "quickening," can feel like flutters, bubbles, or gentle taps. It's an exciting milestone that helps you and your partner connect with your growing baby.

- **Visible baby bump**: By the fourth month, your partner's baby bump is likely becoming more noticeable. Her uterus has grown enough to rise above her pelvic bone, and her abdomen will start to round out. She may need to start wearing maternity clothes for comfort and support.

- **Changes in her body**: She may continue to experience pregnancy symptoms such as morning sickness, fatigue, and breast tenderness, although these symptoms often lessen during the fourth month. Her hormones are stabilizing, and she may feel a surge in energy and an improved sense of well-being.

- **Emotional well-being:** Pregnancy can bring about a range of emotions. Some women feel a sense of relief and increased excitement as they enter the second trimester. In contrast, others may still experience mood swings or anxiety. She needs to prioritize self-care, seek support from loved ones, and discuss any concerns with her healthcare provider.

Weeks 13 and 14

Fundamental changes are happening not only to the mother but to the baby as well. During weeks 13-14 of pregnancy, the second trimester is well underway, and your baby continues to grow and develop. Here's what typically happens during this stage:

- **Size and appearance:** By week 13, your baby is approximately 3 inches (7.6 centimeters) long, about the size of a peach. They will grow to around 4-4.5 inches (10-11.4 centimeters) by week 14. At this point, the baby's body looks more proportional, with the head becoming less dominant.
- **Facial features:** During these weeks, your baby's facial features become more distinct. Their eyes are closer together, and the ears are shifting to their final position on the sides of the head. Eyebrows and eyelashes form, giving the face a more human-like appearance.
- **Limb development:** The limbs continue to develop and gain strength. Your baby can move their arms and legs, although these movements are still uncoordinated. The tiny fingers and toes are more defined, and the nails start to develop.
- **Internal organ growth:** The baby's internal organs are undergoing rapid development. The kidneys produce urine, and the digestive system works as the intestines move from the umbilical cord into the abdomen. The vocal cords are forming, setting the foundation for your baby's ability to make sounds in the future.
- **Lanugo and vernix:** By week 14, a fine hair called lanugo starts to cover your baby's body. This hair helps to protect the skin and is usually shed before birth. Additionally, a waxy substance called vernix caseosa forms, which serves as a protective layer on the skin.
- **Sucking and swallowing:** Your baby's sucking reflex develops more during these weeks. They may suck their thumb or practice swallowing amniotic fluid. This

helps their oral muscles develop and prepares them for feeding after birth.

- **Movement:** While your partner may not feel it, your baby moves and makes small, jerky movements. They flex and extend their limbs, bend their elbows and knees, and move their fingers and toes. These movements are essential for muscle development and coordination.

Weeks 15 and 16

It's important to note that every baby develops at their own pace, and individual experiences may vary. You will get the best insight into how your baby progresses through regularly scheduled screenings and ultrasounds. This is a crucial stage of the pregnancy, and your obstetrician might schedule ultrasounds at a more frequent pace. This is because the baby grows more rapidly, and changes occur faster. When you enter the 15th and 16th weeks of pregnancy, more changes will appear. Here's what usually happens at this time:

- **Size and appearance:** By week 15, your baby is around 4 inches (10 centimeters) long and weighs approximately 2.5 ounces (70 grams). By week 16, your baby grows to about 4.5-5 inches (11-13 centimeters) and weighs around 3.5 ounces (100 grams). It is starting to look more like a miniature human with a rounded body and more defined features.
- **Muscle and bone development:** Your baby's muscles strengthen and develop more during this stage. They

are practicing movements, such as flexing their arms and legs and kicking, although she still may not yet feel them. Their bones are also hardening as they continue to form.

- **Skin and hair:** Your baby's skin is becoming less transparent and more opaque as fat deposits develop underneath. Fine hair called lanugo still covers their body, and a white, waxy substance called the vernix caseosa is present on their skin. The hair and this waxy substance helps to protect and nourish your baby's delicate skin.

- **Facial features:** By this stage, your baby's face is becoming more defined. Their eyes, ears, and nose are in their proper positions. Their lips are formed, and may even be seen sucking their thumb or fingers on ultrasound images. Their facial expressions are more evident as their facial muscles continue to develop.

- **Sensory development:** Your baby's senses are developing further. Their taste buds are forming, and they may be able to taste the amniotic fluid. Their ears are becoming more sensitive, and they can hear sounds from within your body, such as your partner's heartbeat and digestive sounds.

- **Digestive system:** The digestive system of your baby is becoming more functional. Their intestines grow longer and absorb small amounts of sugar from swallowed amniotic fluid. The production of meconium, the first bowel movement, starts in the intestines.

- **Sex development:** If you have an ultrasound during weeks 15-16, it may be possible to determine the baby's gender. However, it's important to note that sometimes it can still be challenging to determine accurately, depending on the baby's position and other factors. Your healthcare provider can provide more information and guidance regarding gender determination.

Weeks 17 through 20

The fifth month of pregnancy, from weeks 17 to 20, is exciting as your baby grows and develops. During this stage, you and your partner may feel more pronounced movements as your baby becomes more active. Their senses are developing, and they may be able to hear sounds from the outside world. Your baby's body is becoming more proportionate, and its skin is thickening. By the end of the fifth month, your baby is typically around 6-7 inches (15-18 centimeters) long and weighs approximately 10-12 ounces (283-340 grams). Your partner may experience a boost in energy and a sense of well-being as they enter the second half of their pregnancy journey. It's necessary to continue attending prenatal check-ups, eat a balanced diet, and take care of your overall health and well-being during this stage.

Between weeks 17 and 20, your baby is "taking shape," becoming more and more proportionate and formed. Here is a summary of these changes:

- **Size and appearance:** By week 17, your baby will be around 5.1 inches (13 centimeters) long and weighs about 5.9 ounces (168 grams). By week 20, they grow to about 6.5-10.2 inches (16-26 centimeters) in length and weigh approximately 10.6 ounces (300 grams). Your baby's body is becoming more proportionate, and its skin is less transparent as fat stores develop underneath.
- **Movement**: As your baby's muscles and nervous system continue to mature, their movements become more pronounced. Your partner may feel distinct flutters, kicks, and rolls as your baby becomes more active. These movements are essential for their muscle and skeletal development.
- **Facial features:** Your baby's facial features become more refined during this stage. Their eyebrows and eyelashes are growing, and their eyes, ears, and nose are appropriately positioned. Their mouth can open and close, and their tooth buds are forming beneath their gums.
- **Sensory development**: By week 20, your baby's senses are developing further. They can hear sounds outside the womb, including your voices and other environmental noises. This is an excellent time to start talking, singing, or playing music for your baby, as they may respond to familiar sounds.

- **Organ development:** By this stage, most of your baby's organs are fully formed and continue to mature. Their digestive system is developing, and their intestines are starting to absorb small amounts of sugar from swallowed amniotic fluid. The lungs are also growing, preparing for breathing outside the womb.
- **Sex determination:** Between weeks 18 and 20, an ultrasound may determine the baby's gender more accurately. Sometimes it can still be challenging to figure out, depending on the baby's position and other factors.
- **Maternal changes:** Your partner's abdomen expands as the baby grows, and she may have a noticeable baby bump. She might also experience pregnancy symptoms like backaches, indigestion, and round ligament pain. Maintaining regular prenatal check-ups and communicating concerns or discomfort with your healthcare provider is important.

Weeks 21 through 24

The sixth month of pregnancy, which spans from weeks 21 to 24, is an equally important time as your baby grows and develops. Your baby's movements become more pronounced at this stage, and you may feel their kicks and wiggles - this time in earnest! Their senses are developing even further, and they can hear sounds outside the womb. Your baby's brain is rapidly evolving, and its lungs are beginning to mature. Your partner may notice physical changes such as an expanding belly and weight gain. Keep attending regular prenatal check-ups and communicate any concerns with your healthcare provider.

The sixth month brings new developments and exciting milestones in your pregnancy journey. And needless to say, it is already a significant stage of pregnancy. Just three more months and your baby will arrive in this world. How exciting! It is a thrilling time full of excitement and anticipation. Both you and your partner will feel those unmistakable butterflies in your stomach whenever you think about birth being just around the corner. Here is what happens with your baby during this time:

- **Size and appearance:** By week 21, your baby will be around 10.5 inches (27 centimeters) long and weigh approximately 12.7 ounces (360 grams). By week 24, they grow to about 11.8 inches (30 centimeters) in length and weigh roughly 1.3 pounds (590 grams). Their body is becoming more proportional as they are gaining more baby fat.
- **Movement:** Your baby's movements become more coordinated and robust during this stage. You may feel kicks, rolls, and somersaults as they explore the space in the womb. These movements are a positive sign of their healthy development and can be felt more distinctly by you.
- **Sensory development:** Your baby's senses continue to develop. They can hear distinct sounds, including your voice and other external noises. They may even respond to familiar sounds or music. Their eyelids have

formed, and their eyes are light-sensitive, although their vision is still developing.

- **Lung development:** Although their lungs are not fully mature, they develop vital structures. The air sacs, known as alveoli, form, and surfactant, a substance that helps the lungs inflate and function correctly, is produced. These developments prepare your baby for breathing independently after birth.

- **Brain growth:** Your baby's brain continues to develop rapidly. The nerve cells are multiplying, and the connections between them are forming. The brain's surface, called the cerebral cortex, is becoming more complex, setting the foundation for future cognitive and sensory processing abilities.

- **Maternal changes:** As your baby grows, your partner will experience physical changes in her body. Her belly continues to expand as the uterus rises higher in the abdomen. Your wife may notice weight gain, and her breasts may become larger and more sensitive. Some common pregnancy symptoms like backaches, leg cramps, and heartburn may persist.

- **Prenatal care:** Regular prenatal check-ups with your healthcare provider are essential during this stage. They will monitor mom's health, check her blood pressure, and may perform additional tests or ultrasounds to assess your baby's growth and well-being. These appointments offer an opportunity to address concerns and ensure a healthy pregnancy.

FINDING OUT YOUR BABY'S SEX

It is around this time that couples usually discover the sex of their baby through various methods, such as ultrasound or genetic testing. If you don't want to be surprised with your baby's sex when the time comes, you will certainly be given the option of finding out. By the second trimester, your baby's genitals are usually developed enough to be identified through ultrasound imaging. The external genitalia becomes more distinguishable, making it easier for healthcare professionals to determine the baby's sex with greater accuracy. This is why many couples opt to find out during this time. The choice, however, is all up to you. There are pros and cons to discovering your baby's sex. Here are the positive aspects of it:

- **Bonding and preparation**: Knowing the sex of the baby can help parents develop a stronger emotional connection with their unborn child. It allows them to envision their future with a specific gender in mind, leading to bonding and attachment. It also enables parents to make practical preparations, such as decorating the nursery, choosing appropriate clothing, and selecting sex-specific names.
- **Emotional and psychological preparation:** Understanding the baby's sex in advance can help parents mentally and emotionally prepare for their child's arrival. It allows them to explore their expectations, dreams, and aspirations for their child, and it can help them adjust their mindset and anticipate the unique experiences associated with raising a boy or

a girl. Say you always wanted a baby boy. You keep the sex a secret, only to discover it's a baby girl. All your dreams suddenly dissipate. That's why it is good to know beforehand, having ample time to prepare and readjust your mindset. It's all-natural.

- **Personal satisfaction:** For some parents, knowing the sex of the baby provides a sense of fulfillment and curiosity satisfaction. It adds an exciting element to their pregnancy journey and enables them to share the news with family and friends. After all, most parents are dying to find out their baby's sex as soon as possible. All that curiosity and anticipation make the wait even harder.

But, wherever there are pros, there are cons too. While finding out the sex at this time is common, some negative aspects still need to be acknowledged. Here are some examples:

- **Surprise element:** Some couples prefer to keep the baby's sex a surprise until birth, cherishing the excitement and anticipation of not knowing. It adds an element of mystery and surprise to the birthing experience. Revealing your baby's sex around the sixth month can ruin that surprise for you. If this is your choice, let your healthcare provider know they should not reveal this.
- **Disappointment or sex preference:** In some cases, parents may have a preference for the sex of their baby, and learning that the baby's sex doesn't align with it can lead to disappointment or sadness. It's essential to

approach sex openly and embrace your child's uniqueness, regardless of sex. Ultimately, it is your baby, child, and cherished offspring. You will adore them nonetheless.

- **Gender stereotypes:** Knowing the baby's sex ahead of time can unintentionally reinforce societal gender stereotypes. Parents may feel pressured to conform to traditional gender norms regarding clothing, toys, and activities. It's important to remember that every child is an individual, and their interests and likings may not align with societal expectations.

As a caring expectant father, you, too, will feel the excitement of the nearing birth. After all, just three months more are left. However, you must be there for your better half to provide support and care. Let's face it, that baby bump is getting much more prominent, and being pregnant is not easy work. Nature has it all arranged: your partner is there to carry the baby - she is the vessel in which life blooms and blossoms. And you are there to offer protection, to provide all that is needed, and to care for her in every way. It is the majesty of life and the sublime balance of all things. Understand your role and cherish it. But above all, understand what your wife is going through. It might be obscure, so we are here to give you a solid insight.

Overall, the second trimester is often considered the most comfortable and enjoyable for many pregnant women. It still doesn't mean it's easy. Here are some of the main things a pregnant woman might experience during this time:

- **Physical changes:** During the second trimester, many early pregnancy symptoms, such as nausea and fatigue, tend to subside or lessen. Women often experience a surge of energy, increased appetite, and general well-being. The uterus expands, causing the belly to grow, and the woman may notice weight gain. Her breasts may also continue to enlarge and become more sensitive as they prepare for breastfeeding.

- **Emotional well-being:** With the relief from early pregnancy discomforts, many women experience improved mood and emotional well-being during the second trimester. Hormonal fluctuations tend to stabilize, reducing mood swings and heightened emotions. This period may bring a sense of excitement and anticipation as the baby's movements become more noticeable, fostering a stronger emotional connection between the mother and her unborn child.

- **Increased sex drive:** Here's one you might enjoy learning about! Many women experience an increase in libido during the second trimester. The hormonal changes, reduced nausea, and increased blood flow to the pelvic area can contribute to heightened sexual desire and pleasure. Communicating with your partner is essential to ensure you both are on the same page about having sex.

- **Body changes and body image:** As your partner's belly grows and the pregnancy progresses, women may have mixed feelings about their changing bodies and body image. Some may embrace the physical changes as a beautiful reminder of the growing life within them. In contrast, others may struggle with body image concerns or body confidence. It can be helpful to seek support from loved ones and engage in self-care practices that promote body positivity and self-acceptance. As a caring partner, don't hesitate to provide compliments and raise the spirits of your loved one.

- **Backaches and discomfort:** As the baby grows, the additional weight can strain your partner's back and cause discomfort. Hormonal changes and relaxation of ligaments can also contribute to backaches and joint pain. Maintaining good posture, wearing supportive shoes, and practicing gentle exercises or prenatal yoga can help alleviate these discomforts.
- **Screening and prenatal care:** Prenatal screenings are necessary during the 2nd trimester. Women will undergo routine prenatal check-ups, including blood tests, ultrasounds, and screenings for genetic conditions. These appointments help monitor the baby's growth and development, as well as the overall health of the pregnant woman.

Sometimes, pregnancy isn't a straightforward and hassle-free process, even after the challenging initial first months have passed. Even at the six-month mark, complications can happen. They are not often, but they are still a possibility. That is why we need to mention them as well. Complications can vary in severity, and healthcare professionals should evaluate each case individually. Here are a few examples of complications that may occur:

- **Gestational diabetes:** Gestational diabetes is a condition that affects some pregnant women and can lead to high blood sugar levels. It is caused by hormonal changes during pregnancy that affect how the body processes sugar in the blood. Treatment usually involves dietary changes, monitoring blood sugar levels, and sometimes medication.
- **Placenta previa:** Placenta previa happens when the placenta partially or completely covers the cervix. It can cause painless vaginal bleeding during the second or third trimester. Treatment depends on the severity of the condition. It may include bed rest, medication, or in more severe cases, a cesarean or C-section delivery.
- **Preterm labor:** Preterm labor refers to the onset of regular contractions and cervical changes before the 37th week of pregnancy. Various factors, such as infections, certain medical conditions, or multiple pregnancies, can cause these contractions. Treatment may involve medication to delay labor, bed rest, or hospitalization to monitor the mother and baby.
- **Miscarriage:** While the risk of miscarriage decreases after the first trimester, it can still occur in the second trimester. Chromosomal abnormalities, infections, or certain medical conditions may cause miscarriage. Treatment depends on the individual situation and may involve increased monitoring and medication; some cases may even require surgery.
- **Preterm premature rupture of membranes (PPROM):** PPROM refers to the break of the amniotic sac before 37 weeks of pregnancy. It can increase the

risk of infection and preterm birth. Treatment may involve bed rest, medication to prevent infection, and sometimes early delivery.

Still, you should not take these complications to heart and worry yourself silly - they are not that common. But you shouldn't disregard them completely, either. Continue to attend regular prenatal check-ups together and communicate any concerns or symptoms with your healthcare provider. These professionals can provide a proper diagnosis, monitor the situation, and determine the most appropriate course of treatment for any complications that may arise. So, don't skimp on your visits to the doctor, and follow all the rules about pregnancy care that you usually do.

HOW TO A.C.E. THE SECOND TRIMESTER!

Acing the second trimester is all about *support*. An expectant father, a first-time dad, a pillar one can rely on, a loved husband or boyfriend - these are your titles, and you should wear them with pride! But you have to earn them as well. So, to A.C.E. the second trimester, be *aware* of your role, *connect* with it, and fully *embrace* it. Gone are the bachelor days. You are now an expectant father and a husband - so A.C.E. it!

Awareness:

You can support your partner during this period in several ways. Your support and your involvement are crucial for their well-being and the health of the baby as well. One of the foremost things you can do during this time is to emphasize the importance of accompanying your partner to prenatal check-ups and antenatal classes. Doing just this shows your involvement and support in your partner's pregnancy journey, and you will be greatly appreciated. It also allows you to stay informed and aware of the progress of the pregnancy, ask questions, and share the experience.

Antenatal classes, also known as prenatal or childbirth education classes, are designed to provide expectant parents with valuable information and skills to navigate pregnancy, childbirth, and early parenthood. Attending these classes can offer numerous benefits, including

education, support, new connections, and practical demonstrations. These classes cover many topics, including pregnancy health, labor, delivery, pain management techniques, breast-feeding, newborn care, and postpartum recovery. They will provide you with the knowledge and skills to make informed decisions and feel more confident throughout the pregnancy.

And you don't just learn the traditional way - you get to try it yourself! These classes often include practical demonstrations of breathing exercises, relaxation techniques, and baby care practices. These hands-on activities help you develop practical skills that can be invaluable during labor, birth, and early parenting. You'd be surprised how quickly you can master the basics and how important they will be later down the road. This will boost your confidence as a first-time dad and show your partner how dedicated you are to her and your baby.

Connection:

You won't be the only couple in these antenatal classes. You will meet other expectant parents, share experiences, and build a support network. Connecting with others going through similar experiences can be reassuring and provide ongoing support during the journey. You're certainly not alone in this!

Pregnancy can bring about various physical and emotional changes for your partner. Be an attentive listener and create an open space for them to express their feelings, concerns, and joys. Effective communication helps you understand their needs better and strengthens your connection as a couple. Don't be a closed book with zero interests. Take the lead, and show you care. You should also take the initiative to learn about pregnancy, the changes your partner is experiencing, and your baby's development during the second trimester. Understanding the process will enable you to provide informed support and engage in meaningful discussions about the pregnancy.

Another important thing is to be involved in matters related to your soon-to-come child. Actively participate in discussions about birth plans, baby names, and other important decisions. Show your interest and involvement in decision-making and respect your partner's preferences and desires. Last but not least is the importance of displaying your love and kindness towards the mother of your child. Pregnancy is emotional, and your partner needs to feel loved and appreciated. Express your affection, gratitude, and admiration for the incredible journey they are going through.

Remember that support isn't just emotional. It is physical as well. Your partner may experience physical discomfort as the pregnancy progresses, making every task challenging. Offer to help with household chores, lift heavy objects, or assist with tasks that may be challenging for them. Providing physical support shows your care and consideration for their well-being. Forget those aged gender roles - take care of the dishes, do the laundry, carry in all the groceries, and scrub that toilet clean.

Embrace:

Still, the bulk of the support you'll have to do is emotional. Pregnancy can bring a range of feelings and emotions to the woman, including excitement, anxiety, and mood swings. Be patient, understanding, and empathetic toward your partner's emotional state. Offer reassurance and positive affirmations, and provide stability and comfort during times of stress or worry. Remind your partner to prioritize self-care activities such as proper nutrition, exercise (as approved by their health-care provider), rest, and relaxation. Offer to join them in activities like prenatal yoga or walks to promote physical and emotional well-being.

With the "moment" quickly approaching, you should prepare and properly welcome your child into this world. And, as we learned thus far, preparation comes in many different shapes and sizes. But how else do you get prepared for a baby?

PREPARING YOUR NURSERY

Another crucial step you should tackle at this time is the preparation of the nursery. It is the little special nook that will be reserved for your baby! You can choose an entire room or devote a small part of your bedroom for this. Creating a nurturing and safe space for your baby is integral to being ready for those first few weeks with your child. Decide on the nursery's location and determine what furniture and items you'll need, such as a crib, changing table, storage, and comfortable seating. Make a checklist of essential baby items and start gathering them gradually. Some things will be optional early on, like complex toys and such. Just the basics will do - a place to sleep, to be safe, and to be dressed and cleaned.

You can ensure the nursery is a safe environment for your baby by "baby-proofing" it. Install outlet covers, secure furniture to the walls, use corner protectors, and remove any potential hazards. Consider installing smoke detectors and baby monitors as well. Some of these will only be necessary once your baby starts crawling and exploring, but no harm in installing them early on. You can also create a welcoming and comforting atmosphere by choosing a color scheme, adding wall decals, hanging curtains, and selecting bedding. Personalize the space with photographs, artwork, or meaningful decorations. This, of course, depends on the sex of your baby. It may be tough to appropriately decorate the room if you still do not know the baby's sex. Remember, however, that babies - after those first few weeks - require visual stimulation through bright and merry colors, joyful images, plush comforting toys, and such. Don't hesitate to decorate in a cute and colorful way!

The last step of preparing your nursery is *storage*. As you enter into parenthood, you will quickly realize that you need a lot of that! Set up storage solutions for baby clothes, diapers, wipes, and other necessities. Create designated spaces for items to make them easily accessible when needed. There will be a lot of baby-related stuff in your life from now on. Make sure there's plenty of free space for everything.

CREATING A BIRTH PLAN

You should take care of one more thing to truly A.CE. the second trimester: a birth plan. What's that, you might wonder? Well, a birth plan is a written document that outlines your preferences and desires for the labor, delivery, and immediate postpartum period. It is a communication tool between you, your partner, and your healthcare team to ensure your wishes are understood and respected during this critical time. Why is it important to have a birth plan? One of the major advantages of a birth plan is *communication*. A birth plan lets you clearly communicate your preferences, concerns, and expectations to your healthcare providers. It ensures that everyone involved in your care is aware of your desires, promoting open and informed discussions about your birth experience. That way, you are confident everything will go as planned.

Writing a birth plan also empowers you to actively participate in decision-making and take ownership of your birth experience. It encourages you to become informed about different options and make choices that align with your values and preferences. Ultimately, creating a birth plan enables you to explore additional alternatives and interventions available during childbirth. It allows you to consider various scenarios and make contingency plans if your initial preferences are unmet. Writing a birth plan during the second or early third trimester is highly recommended. This allows you enough time to research and discuss your options with your healthcare provider. It's important to remember that birth plans should be flexible and open to adjustments based on the circumstances and medical advice during labor. Here are some things to include in a birth plan:

- **Location of the birthing experience:** Will this take place in a hospital setting, a birth center, or at home? All are viable options with different types of healthcare providers, such as physicians and certified nurse-midwives. We will focus on the hospital setting in chapter five.
- **What your partner's ideal birthing environment looks like:** Does she prefer the lights to be dimmed? Would she like a specific type of music to be playing? Does she want a T.V. to be on? Consider what would make her most comfortable.
- **Who will be present during the actual birth:** Talk about who she wants to be in the room while she is actively giving birth. Besides you (I mean, hopefully, she wants you there) does she want any other loved ones there? Does she want any friends present?
- **What type of pain relief is acceptable for your partner:** Discuss whether or not your partner wants

pain medications such as an epidural or other narcotics during or after the birthing process. She may have specific preferences when it comes to more potent pain medications.

- **Who will cut the umbilical cord:** Physicians frequently allow dads to cut the umbilical cord. Some fathers may not be comfortable with that, so consider this when creating your birth plan.

In this chapter, we delved into the second trimester of pregnancy, a period often marked by increased comfort and excitement for expectant parents. We explored various aspects of this period, including the changes experienced by the pregnant woman, the development of the baby, and the importance of your role in support and preparation. Throughout the second trimester, pregnant women often experience physical and emotional changes. Many find relief from early pregnancy symptoms, regain energy, and may even notice increased sex drive. We emphasized the significance of open communication, understanding, and support from partners to navigate these changes together.

As we move forward, the next chapter will explore the final trimester of pregnancy: the third trimester. This period brings its own unique experiences and challenges as the countdown to meeting your baby draws near. We will delve into the physical changes, emotional preparations, and final steps leading you toward childbirth and parenthood. Join us as we navigate the journey through the third trimester and prepare for the much-anticipated arrival of your little one.

YOU ARE ACEING THIS!

"Fathering is not something perfect men do, but something that perfects the man."

— FRANK PITTMAN

Doesn't it feel like you get over one pregnancy milestone or hurdle, your emotions level out, and then all of a sudden, the next loop of the rollercoaster smacks you in the face out of the blue? You tell yourself that you've got it…until you don't!

Get used to this feeling because this is what being a parent is all about. Your child will take their first steps and you will feel the biggest sense of pride ever. Then they will throw a tantrum that would scare half an army and you wonder where you are going wrong.

The only thing your family needs from you is your best. And everything you learn and put into practice will only make you better.

By taking the effort to discover more about pregnancy and how to be a supportive partner, you are actually doing something else that has a positive impact on a much larger scale.

Previous generations didn't necessarily help the modern man. Dated images of men not being involved in pregnancy have led to strong stereotypes that we are trying to fight. We need to get more men on board and you can help!

By leaving a review on Amazon, you can let other first-time dads know that there is a practical guide to enable them to be the best partner and dads they can be.

Your review will only take a few minutes and in those few minutes, you could change how other men experience pregnancy. Just like you, they need to know that what they are going through is normal and they aren't alone!

Scan the QR codes below for a quick review!

4

THE THIRD TRIMESTER

nd so it happens. As soon as you know it, the *third trimester* is at your doorstep. The very last stretch of your magnificent pregnancy journey. The big three. The big outro - to the big intro. But even though the end of the pregnancy is near, plenty will still occur in these last three months. And we must address all the big happenings and all the major milestones.

CHOOSING A NAME

Your child's name is one of the most important milestones you will tackle in the last three months. Personally, it was one of the most unique and rewarding experiences of pregnancy - the way I experienced it. It's like a final exclamation mark to everything you experienced thus far. *Your child* will have a name. Instantly it becomes a person, a tiny new human entering the grand stage of life.

In the third trimester, you'll find yourself eagerly thinking about a name for your child. So many possibilities! Each one sounds unique, and you want to choose carefully. After all, the name remains with us for a lifetime. So it has to be good. Some parents, however, decide not to select a name for their child even in the third trimester. But for most couples, it is the ideal time. And here are some reasons why you *should* choose a baby name in the third trimester:

- **Emotional connection:** You may feel a stronger emotional connection to your baby as the due date approaches. Choosing a name allows you to envision your child as an individual, fostering a deeper bond with them even before birth. Say, for example, you select *James* as the name for your baby. Instantly you think: *"James is coming! Who is James? What kind of person will he be?"*
- **Time for research and reflection:** The third trimester provides ample time for researching and reflecting on potential names. It's an excellent opportunity to explore different options, meanings, cultural significance, and family traditions associated with names. Here's a chance to reflect on your ancestors, grandparents, and great-grandparents. You may find inspiration there!
- **Shared decision-making:** Involving both partners in choosing a name can strengthen your bond and ensure you feel included in this crucial decision. It's a chance to discuss your preferences, consider each other's suggestions, and find a name that resonates with both of you. For example, I wanted to name my first

daughter Isabella. In contrast, my wife wanted to choose a name related to stars and the galaxy. We compromised and named her Stella, which resonated well with both of us.

There are several things to consider when choosing a name for your baby. Again, the choice you make will stick with your child for a lifetime, so don't choose anything silly, like *Khaleesi* or *Anakin.* Make the name meaningful, beautiful, and unique. Think of your child in their youth - and how their name would sound to them and to others. Explore the meanings and origins of names to find something special to you and your partner. It could be a name that represents your cultural heritage, has a positive connotation, or carries a personal meaning for you and your partner. Pay attention to the sound and compatibility of the name with your last name. Consider how the full name will flow together and if it sounds pleasing to your ears.

Another thing you may consider is family traditions or cultural naming practices that you may want to honor. It can be a way to pay homage to your heritage or to name your baby after a beloved family member. Also, consider how others may perceive the name throughout your child's life. Consider factors such as potential nicknames, pronunciation, and any associations that may arise. One of the best ways to "test out" your baby's potential name is by saying it out loud. Say the name and imagine calling your child - just like that. Sometimes hearing the name spoken aloud can help you determine if it feels right for your baby. At times, it just makes sense - at others, it does not. If potential names don't seem right, try finding some inspiration. Explore different sources of motivation, such as books, movies, historical figures, or nature. These sources can spark ideas and help you discover unique and meaningful names. Trust your instincts and choose a name that feels right for your baby. Remember, it's a decision that will stay with your child throughout their life, so follow your heart and choose a name that brings you joy and resonates with your family. And sometimes, a name feels *right*, no matter what.

THE IMPORTANCE OF SOCIAL SUPPORT IN PREGNANCY

No one is on the pregnancy journey entirely alone. There is your partner by your side, but even then, you might sometimes feel overwhelmed and clueless. And even then - *you are not alone.* Especially if you have people around you, a social network of supporters and connections. After all, social connection plays a vital role in our overall well-being, which also holds true during pregnancy. And maintaining these social connections can have numerous benefits for expectant parents. A solid social network provides emotional support during the ups and downs of pregnancy. Sharing your experiences, fears, and joys with friends, family, or other expectant parents can alleviate stress and provide a sense of comfort. Likewise, social connections offer a space to find validation and understanding. Connecting with others going through a similar journey allows you to share everyday experiences, exchange advice, and gain reassurance that you're not alone in your feelings and challenges.

Your connections provide a valuable source of information and resources. Fellow parents or experienced individuals can offer insights, recommendations, and practical tips that can be beneficial during pregnancy and as you prepare for parenthood. It's great having a couple that recently entered parenthood in your social circle - they can give you a great deal of valuable information and support for you and your partner's pregnancy journey.

Most importantly, these relationships offer a powerful sense of belonging, and you can build a proper little community of parents and expectant parents. Being part of such a supportive network where you can celebrate milestones, share stories, and receive encouragement enhances your overall well-being and helps combat feelings of isolation.

These social connections can vary, depending on your lifestyle, family, and the size of your friend circle. Your circle may include family, friends, acquaintances from prenatal classes, pregnancy support groups, and online communities. A friendly voice and supportive embrace can mean so much when pressures rise. Another positive aspect of having supportive friends is that they can be there for the pregnant mother while you are at work, for instance.

There are numerous ways to find and expand your social connections. Don't be shy; meeting new people and creating new and lasting friendships is never too late. Here are a few tips to follow:

- **Seek out existing networks:** Identify existing social networks, such as friends who are already parents or family members who have gone through pregnancy. Reach out to them, express your desire for support, and nurture those connections.
- **Attend prenatal classes or support groups:** Enroll in prenatal classes or join support groups specifically designed for expectant parents. These settings provide opportunities to meet others who are going through similar experiences and establish supportive relationships.
- **Join online communities:** Explore online platforms dedicated to pregnancy and parenting. Participate in discussions, ask questions, and share your own experiences. Building connections online can provide a valuable source of support and information.
- **Communicate openly:** Initiate conversations with other expectant parents in person or online. Share your experiences, ask for advice, and offer support to others. Open and honest communication is the foundation for forming strong social connections.
- **Attend local events or workshops:** Look for events or seminars focused on pregnancy or parenting. These events provide opportunities to meet other expectant

parents in your community and build connections outside virtual spaces.

- **Be proactive:** Take the initiative to reach out to other expectant parents or join relevant social groups. Proactively seeking social connections increases the likelihood of forming supportive relationships.

THE CHANGES THAT OCCUR DURING THE THIRD TRIMESTER

The third trimester, the final stage of your pregnancy journey, is when considerable changes continue. The seventh month marks a significant milestone during this period. Your baby's growth continues rapidly at this stage, and its organs are nearly fully developed. Mom may feel the baby's movements more prominently as they become stronger and more frequent. She may also experience increased discomfort as her belly expands, including backaches and shortness of breath. Regular prenatal check-ups become even more crucial to monitor her health and the baby's growth. With each passing day, anticipation grows as you both eagerly prepare for the upcoming arrival of your little one. Here is what happens between weeks 25 and 28:

Baby's Growth and Development:

- By the 25th week, the baby is approximately 9 inches long and weighs around 1.5 pounds. The baby's growth accelerates over the next few weeks, and they continue to mature and develop.

- The baby's lungs continue to develop and mature, producing surfactant, which is a substance that helps the lungs expand and function properly after birth.
- The baby's senses, including hearing and touch, continue to develop and become more refined. They can now respond to external sounds and stimuli.
- The eyes are also undergoing significant changes, with the eyelids becoming more developed and capable of opening and closing.
- The baby's brain continues to grow and develop rapidly, forming complex neural connections in preparation for life outside the womb.

Physical Changes in Your Partner:

- Mom's belly continues to expand, and she may notice an increase in the size of her abdomen as the baby grows.
- Some women may start experiencing Braxton Hicks contractions, irregular and less painful contractions that help prepare the uterus for labor. They are considered normal unless they become regular and more intense.
- As your baby's weight increases, your partner may experience backaches, pelvic pain, and general discomfort due to the strain on the body.
- Fatigue may persist or increase during the seventh month due to hormonal changes and the physical demands of pregnancy. Your partner needs to prioritize rest and self-care.

- The growing uterus puts pressure on her diaphragm, leading to feelings of breathlessness or shortness of breath. Taking breaks, practicing good posture, and avoiding strenuous activities can help manage this symptom.

During the seventh month, regular antenatal check-ups become even more critical. These appointments allow healthcare providers to monitor the mother's health, check the baby's growth, and address any concerns or questions. It's also crucial for both expectant parents to begin finalizing birth plans, preparing for labor and delivery, and considering any necessary preparations for the postpartum period.

By the eighth month, your wife's belly will undoubtedly be large. The size of her stomach can depend on many factors. Regardless, it will definitely be a reminder that the *big day* is coming closer! Between weeks 29 and 30, your baby will continue its rapid growth. Here are the changes happening during this period:

Baby's Growth and Development:

- By week 29, the baby measures around 15 inches in length and weighs approximately 2.5 to 3 pounds.
- The baby's brain continues developing rapidly, forming intricate neural connections.
- The baby's lungs are further maturing as they produce increasing amounts of surfactant.

- The baby's eyes are becoming more developed, and they can distinguish between light and darkness. However, their vision will still be blurry at birth.
- The baby's immune system is strengthened as they receive essential antibodies from the mother, which provide some level of protection against infections after birth.

Physical Changes in Your Partner:

As the third trimester progresses, the mother may experience various physical changes and pregnancy symptoms, which are essentially the same as in the previous month.

- The mother's abdomen continues to expand, and she may notice increased discomfort due to the pressure on her organs and ligaments.
- As the uterus expands upward, it puts pressure on the diaphragm, leading to continued feelings of breathlessness.
- The Braxton Hicks contractions, as mentioned above, may become more noticeable and frequent during this time. Again, these irregular contractions help prepare the uterus for labor but shouldn't be unbearable.
- The growing baby and uterus can put pressure on the bladder, causing the mother to urinate more frequently.
- Some women may experience swelling, particularly in the hands, feet, and ankles. Elevating the legs, staying hydrated, and avoiding prolonged periods of standing can help reduce swelling.

Regular prenatal check-ups continue to closely monitor the mother's health and the baby's growth. These appointments may include checking the baby's position, measuring the uterus, monitoring blood pressure, and addressing any concerns or questions.

Another thing that could occur at this time is *nesting*. As a matter of fact, many expectant parents experience a proper surge in nesting instincts during this period. It's common to have the urge to clean, organize the home, and make final preparations for your baby's arrival. Nesting can include setting up the nursery, washing baby clothes, and ensuring all essential items are ready. This instinct often manifests as an intense need to create a safe, comfortable, and nurturing space for the newborn. After all, you naturally want your child to be safe in a clean and comfortable environment. The nesting instinct is believed to be a natural biological response triggered by hormonal changes and the upcoming due date.

Of course, this instinct does not manifest the same for everyone. If you don't feel the need for these activities or do them as usual, don't think that something's wrong. All of this is perfectly normal.

And so we reach the *fabled* ninth month! This is an incredibly fascinating period - the grand finale. All expectant parents are restless, super excited, and often impatient around this time. These are the final weeks before the baby arrives! Of course, with that being said - you definitely have reasons for excitement. During this time, the baby's growth is nearly complete, and they are preparing for life outside the womb. Here's a quick rundown of the significant developments during this period:

Baby's Growth and Development:

- Your baby is now fully formed, weighing around 6 to 9 pounds on average and measuring approximately 19 to 22 inches long.
- They have developed a layer of fat that helps regulate body temperature after birth.
- The baby's organs, including the lungs, digestive system, and brain, are fully functional and ready for life outside the womb.

Physical Changes in Your Partner:

- Your partner's body continues to undergo changes and prepare for labor and delivery.
- The growing baby puts pressure on the pelvic area, leading to increased discomfort, including backaches, pelvic pain, and frequent urination. This is especially true if your baby happens to be above average in terms of weight and size.
- Braxton Hicks contractions may become more frequent and intense as her body prepares for labor. It's vital to differentiate these contractions from actual labor contractions.
- The physical demands of late-stage pregnancy and increased anticipation can lead to heightened fatigue. Resting and prioritizing self-care becomes even more

critical during this time.

The ninth month is a crucial time for final preparations. Expectant parents may complete the last-minute tasks, such as packing a hospital bag, finalizing birth plans, and ensuring all necessary items are ready for the baby's arrival. It's also an ideal time to discuss last-minute questions or concerns with health-care providers. If you have done everything right thus far, you didn't miss out on something along the way - make sure to leave important things for the very last minute. All in all, the ninth month is a truly memorable period. It is a time of antici-pation, readiness, and immense joy as you and your partner eagerly await the arrival of your little one.

Certain complications can arise during the third trimester of pregnancy, requiring medical attention. Here's a brief overview of some common complications (some of which we have explained previously but will explain again), their causes, and possible treatments:

- **Gestational diabetes:** Gestational diabetes is a condition that affects some pregnant women and can lead to high blood sugar levels. It is caused by hormonal changes during pregnancy that affect how the body processes sugar in the blood. Treatment usually involves dietary changes, monitoring blood sugar levels, and sometimes medication.
- **Pre-eclampsia**: Pre-eclampsia is characterized by high blood pressure and damage to organs, such as the liver and kidneys. The exact cause is unknown, but it is

believed to involve problems with the development of the placenta. Treatment may involve close monitoring, bed rest, medication to manage blood pressure, and, in severe cases, early delivery of the baby.

- **Placenta previa:** Placenta previa happens when the placenta partially or completely covers the cervix. This can cause bleeding. The exact cause is unclear, but it may be related to the position and development of the placenta. Treatment depends on the severity and may involve bed rest, close monitoring, and sometimes, delivery by cesarean section.
- **Preterm labor:** Preterm labor is the onset of regular contractions and cervical changes before 37 weeks of pregnancy. Causes can include infections, uterine abnormalities, or certain lifestyle factors. Treatment may involve medication to stop or delay labor, bed rest, and interventions to promote the baby's lung development.
- **Growth restrictions:** Fetal growth restrictions occur when the baby's growth is significantly below average. Causes can include placental problems, maternal health conditions, or genetic factors. Treatment may involve increased monitoring, ultrasound assessments, and, in severe cases, early delivery.
- **Stillbirth:** Stillbirth is the loss of a baby after the 20th week of pregnancy. Causes can vary and may include problems with the placenta, genetic abnormalities, infections, or complications with the umbilical cord. Treatment involves the delivery of the baby and emotional support for the parents.

It's important to note that while these complications can occur, they are not inevitable for every pregnancy. Regular prenatal care and open communication with healthcare providers are essential for monitoring and addressing potential complications. Early detection and appropriate management can significantly improve outcomes for both the mother and the baby.

This final stage of pregnancy can bring its own challenges, and it becomes crucial for expectant partners to be aware of each other's mental, emotional, and physical well-being. It is a time when the mother may experience increased discomfort, fatigue, and heightened emotions. By being attuned and supportive, partners can provide the necessary care and help alleviate some burdens. However, balancing work and personal life can be demanding, and sometimes it may feel overwhelming to fulfill all responsibilities. In such situations, seeking help from family or friends is essential. Don't hesitate to ask for assistance with household chores, running errands, or simply lending a listening ear. Even small gestures of support can make a significant difference in relieving stress and promoting overall well-being.

Remember, being present for your partner helps them feel supported and strengthens your bond as a couple. Offering empathy, understanding, and reassurance can go a long way in creating a positive and nurturing environment during this critical phase of pregnancy. Prioritize open communication, make time for quality moments together, and seek professional help if needed.

HOW TO A.C.E. THE THIRD TRIMESTER!

Tick, tock! The time approaches when your baby will finally arrive into the world! As a father-to-be, you will have plenty of responsibilities in this final month. At this time, your partner will need your support more than ever before! To successfully A.C.E. the third trimester, you must keep on your toes!

Awareness:

To help your partner, you should support her in every way possible. She will certainly know to appreciate all your efforts. When she's nine months pregnant, you must be aware that many things become challenging for her. Feel free to help with basic daily tasks, such as household chores, lifting heavy objects, or reaching difficult-to-access areas. Offer to give them a soothing massage or foot rub to relieve any discomfort they may be experiencing. Sometimes, even the most minor things can go a long way! Make that midnight ice cream run!

As I have said before, support is not just physical - it is emotional, too. And it should be provided by you from your partner's first day of pregnancy - up to the very last. Offer reassurance and remind your partner that you are there to support them through this journey. Be kind and understanding, fun and optimistic. Be the safe space that she needs in times of worry and tiredness.

Of course, this also includes going to the prenatal check-ups, appointments, and classes - if you have the option, do not leave your partner to attend these all on her own. Your company and involvement are crucial in the ninth month of pregnancy.

THE HOSPITAL BAG

The hospital bag is another vital step to cover to truly A.C.E. the third trimester. As the due date approaches, it's critical to have a hospital bag prepared and ready for when the time comes to go to the hospital for labor and delivery. Here are some essentials to include in the hospital bag during the ninth month:

- **Clothing**: Pack comfortable and loose-fitting clothes for both you and your partner. This may include pajamas, a robe, underwear, socks, and slippers. Remember to pack a going-home outfit for the baby as well.
- **Toiletries**: Include toiletries such as a toothbrush, toothpaste, shampoo, conditioner, soap, and any other personal care items you may need. Consider packing items for postpartum care, such as nursing pads and maternity pads for your partner.
- **Important documents:** Bring your identification, health insurance information, and any necessary hospital paperwork. If you created one together, having a copy of your birth plan is also a good idea.
- **Electronics and entertainment:** Bring chargers for your phone, camera, or other electronic devices. You can capture special moments during labor and after the baby's arrival. Consider packing books, magazines, or

other forms of entertainment to help pass the time during the birthing process.

- **Snacks and drinks:** Pack some snacks and drinks to energize you and your partner during the birthing process. Opt for healthy, easy-to-digest options like granola bars, fruit, or nuts. Check with the hospital about any food restrictions they may have.
- **Comfort items**: Include items that provide comfort and relaxation, such as a pillow, a favorite blanket, or a soothing essential oil or aromatherapy diffuser. The dreaded hospital dad "bed," usually a recliner or small bench, might be all you get to sleep on, so keep this in mind and prepare to sleep uncomfortably.
- **Baby essentials:** Pack items for the baby, including diapers, wipes, baby clothes, and a blanket. Invest in an infant car seat, as your hospital will require it for a safe ride home.

Of course, the essentials you'll have to bring along can depend on the hospital, country, and standard practices in your area. Keeping in close contact with your obstetrician, you will know what is necessary to bring along when the time comes.

You should do some preparation at home as well. When your baby arrives, the first few days - or weeks - could be hectic, and you may sometimes be tied up at home. For these reasons, stocking up on food, basic necessities, and baby-related items is a good idea. You will feel much better prepared if you have everything you need - close at hand.

Another critical part of pre-birth preparation is to be ready to get your partner to the hospital when the time comes. Sometimes, birth can come unexpectedly, and you must be prepared to act whenever that happens. A great piece of advice is familiarizing yourself with the route. Depending on where you live, the hospital could be far away. And if you are a driver (which is a nifty thing to be when you become a parent), you will have to bring your partner to the hospital. Study Google Maps, find the best route to the hospital, and take one afternoon to drive there yourself and memorize the way. Getting to the hospital safely and without hiccups will be a great advantage.

Connection:

During the final days of the third trimester, it will be crucial that your partner (and you) remain calm, stress-free, and laid back. You both should get plenty of rest at this time. Make sure your home is cozy and tidy, eliminate all causes of stress, and engage in some fun, relaxing activities. Adopt a positive, merry attitude and stick to it - no matter what. An excellent way for the two of you to unwind and recharge your batteries is a fun date night. It could be one of the last ones for a while, so make it memorable and make it count. You can use this date night to strengthen your bond, revisit the past, and rekindle the flame of love that connects you. Revisit your first date, the moment you met, or your marriage and travel adventures. It's great to unwind and forget about everything - once in a while.

Choosing a pediatrician is one of the last essential things you should take care of before birth. Having a pediatrician in place before childbirth ensures continuity of care for your baby. Once your little one arrives, you'll have a trusted healthcare professional familiar with your family's medical history that can provide consistent, comprehensive care from the very beginning. Moreover, knowing that you have a pediatrician lined up can give you peace of mind when there are already so many things to think about. It eliminates the added stress of finding a pediatrician right after childbirth when you may be tired and overwhelmed. Pediatricians monitor your baby's growth, development, and overall health. By choosing a pediatrician beforehand, you can schedule well-baby check-ups and ensure your baby receives timely vaccinations and screenings according to the recommended schedule.

When choosing your pediatrician, seek recommendations from trusted sources, such as friends, family, or your obstetrician. They can provide insights based on personal experiences with pediatricians in your area. Schedule a meeting or interview with potential pediatricians to gauge their compatibility with your family's values and preferences. Consider their approach to healthcare, communication style, and willingness to listen and answer questions.

I recommend starting the search for a pediatrician during the second or the third trimester of pregnancy, allowing ample time for research, consultations, and making an informed decision. This way, you can focus on enjoying the early days with your baby, knowing that their healthcare needs are in capable hands.

Embrace:

And so it begins! Just like that, nine months have breezed by, and the three trimesters have passed. You have done so much to support your partner throughout pregnancy and have prepared as much as possible for the arrival of your little one. Please pat yourself on the back, as you have truly earned it. Be proud of yourself as an incredibly involved partner and an expectant father who could be as ready as ever.

As we move forward, the next chapter will explore the highly anticipated moment of childbirth. We will dive into the signs of labor, the stages of labor and delivery, and what to expect during this transformative experience. We will also provide insights into how you can support your partner during labor and embrace the incredible journey of bringing your baby into the world.

5

THE MOMENT YOU'VE BEEN WAITING FOR

The anticipation must be killing you by now! Any day now, your little child will come to the grand stage of life, opening an entirely new episode of your life as a father with its arrival. You are probably burning with anticipation and joy, not knowing what exactly waits around the corner or what life will look like from now on. There could also be fluctuating emotions of worry and fear. But all that is absolutely normal. It is natural to have a thousand questions twirling in your mind.

The due date is one of the first things to mention around this time. What happens if the pregnancy goes *past* this date? If the pregnancy goes past the due date, your doctor may decide to induce labor to ensure the well-being of both the mother and the baby. Reasons for induction are many - they could be due to factors such as prolonged pregnancy, concerns about the baby's health, complications, or the mother's health conditions.

WAYS TO INDUCE LABOR

How will the doctor induce labor? Well, there are different methods used to induce labor. Here are the ones commonly used:

- **Membrane sweeping:** The doctor will use their finger to separate the amniotic sac from the cervix. This will stimulate the release of hormones that can trigger contractions.
- **Medications**: Your doctor may administer medications, such as prostaglandins or oxytocin, to initiate or strengthen contractions.
- **Artificial rupture of membranes:** The doctor may manually break the amniotic sac to start labor.

Make sure to discuss the possibility of labor induction with your doctor. They will be able to answer all your inquiries perfectly. It would help if you also understood the potential side effects of this procedure, such as more intense contractions, the need for pain relief, and the possibility of cesarean delivery. Trust your healthcare team and their expertise to ensure you feel well-informed and supported throughout the induction process.

THE COMMON SIGNS OF LABOR

Of course, as the moment of childbirth comes closer, it would be helpful to familiarize yourself with the common signs of labor. That way, you'll be able to recognize the real contractions and be ready to act at a moment's notice. However, remember that every pregnancy is different, and signs and symptoms might vary from woman to woman. Nevertheless, here are some of the most common signs of labor to look out for in your partner:

- **Regular and increasing contractions:** Contractions are the tightening and relaxing of the uterus. In true labor, contractions become regular, stronger, and closer together over time. They often start in the lower back and radiate to the front of the abdomen. Time the contractions to see if they follow a consistent pattern. When contractions last 45 to 60 seconds and are 5 minutes apart, it's time to call your healthcare provider and head to the hospital for delivery.
- **Bloody show:** A discharge of mucus tinged with blood, often called a "bloody show," may occur as the cervix dilates and effaces (thins out). It is a typical sign that labor is approaching.
- **Water breaking:** The amniotic sac rupture, commonly known as water breaking, can happen as a gush or a slow trickle of fluid. It may be transparent or have a pale yellow or greenish tinge. If your partner's water breaks, it is crucial to contact your healthcare provider, as it is a strong indication that labor is imminent.

- **Back pain and pressure:** Increasing pressure and discomfort in the lower back, similar to menstrual cramps, can signify labor. This discomfort may be accompanied by a feeling of heaviness or pressure in the pelvis.
- **Pelvic pressure and baby's movement:** As the baby descends into the birth canal, your partner may experience increased pelvic pressure and a sensation of the baby "dropping" lower into her abdomen. She may also notice a decrease in the baby's movements as they settle into the optimal birthing position.
- **Nesting instinct:** Women can experience bursts of energy and strong urges to prepare the home for the baby just before labor begins. This nesting instinct can manifest as an intense desire to clean, organize, or complete unfinished tasks.
- **Gastrointestinal changes:** In the days leading up to labor, your partner may experience diarrhea or loose stools. This is the body's way of clearing the bowel to prepare for childbirth.

Remember that these signs can vary from person to person, and not all women will experience the same symptoms or in the same order. If you and your partner notice any of these signs or have concerns about the onset of labor, don't hesitate to contact your healthcare provider. They will guide you and determine whether to go to the hospital or the birthing center. Sometimes it can be tough to differentiate between false and real contractions, so your best bet is to contact your doctor.

Before the time comes, it is a good idea to preregister for your child's birth. This way, you won't have to deal with all the registration paperwork while trying to get your partner into the birthing room simultaneously. You can ignore the emergency room entirely and go straight to the birthing center. Trust me. This will save you so much time and help you skip the anxiety of surprising the hospital with your partner's labor.

Either way, when the time comes - it comes. Most of the time, you *will* know when it's actual labor, and before you know it, you'll be in the hospital. From there on, expectant fathers have an important supportive role. Once you arrive in your hospital room, your job is to help your partner be as comfortable as possible while she is experiencing intense contraction pains. Remember that labor can last up to a few hours and sometimes even longer. My wife's first labor was prolonged and took approximately 27 hours! My experience was a bit extreme, so don't be afraid, as your partner's labor will likely be shorter. Please do your best to hold your partner's hands, help her switch positions, and adjust her pillows. Being present through this phase will strengthen your bond as a couple. Another thing to consider is whether or not you want to present for the grand finale, the actual live birth of your child. The choice is entirely personal.

STAGES OF BIRTH

But in any case, we will go over the basics of *vaginal birth* so that you can know - in a way - the exact process of your baby's entry into the world. Vaginal birth, also known as normal or spontaneous delivery, is the natural process of birth by which a baby is born through the vaginal canal. It usually involves several stages:

- **Stage 1: Early Labor** - During this initial stage, the cervix starts to soften, thin out (efface), and gradually dilate (open). Contractions may begin irregularly and become more frequent, lasting around 30 to 60 seconds. This stage can last for several hours or more.
- **Stage 2: Active Labor** - As the cervix dilates, contractions become more powerful and regular. This stage involves active pushing as the baby moves through the birth canal. The baby's head starts to descend, and with each contraction, the mother actively pushes to help the baby progress. The length of this stage varies, but it typically lasts a few hours.
- **Stage 3: Delivery of the Placenta** - After the baby is born, the uterus continues to contract to expel the placenta (afterbirth). This stage is usually brief and occurs within 10 to 30 minutes after the baby's birth.

Healthcare providers monitor the mother and baby's vital signs throughout the process and provide support and guidance. Pain relief options, such as epidural anesthesia or other medications, may be available depending on the mother's preferences and the healthcare facility's protocols. It's important to note that every birth is unique, and the duration and progression of labor can vary from woman to woman. The healthcare team will closely monitor the progress of labor and make decisions based on the safety and well-being of both the mother and baby.

In some cases, however, due to various reasons, a natural, vaginal birth is not a viable option. When this happens, your doctor could proceed with a C-Section (Cesarean) to deliver the baby safely. This is a surgical procedure in which the baby is delivered through an incision made in your partner's abdomen and uterus. C-Sections are very common. In fact, about 30% of babies in the US are cesarian births. Here's a concise explanation of what a C-Section entails:

- **Anesthesia:** Before the procedure, the mother receives anesthesia, which can be either regional anesthesia (such as epidural or spinal anesthesia) or general anesthesia, depending on the specific circumstances and medical considerations.
- **Incision**: Once the anesthesia takes effect, the surgeon makes an incision in the lower abdomen, typically horizontal along the bikini line (a horizontal incision) or vertical (a vertical incision) in some cases. The incision allows access to the uterus.
- **Uterine Incision and Delivery**: After opening the abdomen, the surgeon makes a cut into the uterus. The type of uterine incision may vary depending on the situation, such as a horizontal (transverse) incision or a

vertical (classical) incision. The baby is then carefully delivered through the uterine incision.

- **Placental Delivery and Closure**: Following the baby's birth, the surgeon removes the placenta from the uterus and examines the incisions to ensure no excessive bleeding. The uterus and abdominal incisions are then closed with stitches or staples.
- **Recovery**: After the procedure, the mother is moved to a recovery area, where her vital signs are monitored, and she is provided with appropriate pain management and post-operative care. The length of hospital stay and recovery time can vary depending on individual circumstances.

A C-Section may need to be planned in advance for medical reasons or performed as an emergency procedure during labor if there are complications or concerns about the mother's or baby's well-being. Usually, a couple will know before delivery that a C-Section needs to be planned. It's important to note that a cesarean section is a surgical procedure carrying certain risks and considerations. The healthcare team decides to perform a C-section based on the best interests of the mother and baby.

YOUR LITTLE ONE IS HERE!

Congratulations! The moment you've so patiently awaited is finally here - the birth of your first child! This is a significant milestone in any person's life, and we know that you are certainly brimming with emotions, feeling proud, accomplished, excited, and thrilled. It's undoubtedly a joyous moment

- filled with wonder, love, and anticipation for the incredible journey ahead. Your lives have been forever changed, and your hearts will soon experience a love like no other before it. So cherish these precious moments as you embark on this beautiful adventure of parenthood.

Before you start celebrating, however, there are a few things to review. You are most likely wondering what happens with your baby once it is delivered:

- **Baby's appearance:** Your baby's skin may initially appear to be blue in color. This is absolutely normal, as their skin will become pink after taking their first breaths outside the womb. Their hands and feet may stay bluish for a few hours. This is also normal. Their skin may also be covered in vernix, blood, and amniotic fluid before being cleaned by the nurses and doctors. Your baby's head may also be shaped like a cone as it had to squish through mom during birth. Their flexible skull should adjust to a more normal shape within the first few days.
- **Apgar assessment:** Within the first few minutes of birth, a healthcare provider performs an Apgar assessment to evaluate the baby's overall well-being. This assessment assigns a score based on the baby's heart rate, breathing, muscle tone, reflexes, and skin color.
- **Cutting the umbilical cord:** The healthcare provider clamps and cuts the umbilical cord, which previously connected the baby to the placenta. This separates the

baby from the placental circulation, and the cord stump (connected to your baby's belly button) is typically left to dry and eventually fall off over the course of a few weeks. Your healthcare provider will often give you, as the father, the opportunity to cut the umbilical cord if you choose to.

- **Clearing the airways:** If necessary, the healthcare provider clears the baby's airways of any mucus or fluids to ensure proper breathing. This may involve suctioning the nose and mouth gently.

- **Skin-to-skin contact:** To promote bonding and regulation of the baby's temperature, healthcare providers place the baby on the mother's chest. This practice has numerous benefits and helps initiate breastfeeding, stabilizes the baby's heart rate, and provides comfort and reassurance.

- **Newborn examination:** Your healthcare provider conducts a thorough physical examination of your baby, checking vital signs, reflexes, and general health. They examine the baby's skin, head, eyes, mouth, heart, lungs, abdomen, and limbs.

- **Administration of preventive measures:** Depending on the hospital's protocols and regional guidelines, the baby may receive specific preventive measures. These commonly include the administration of vitamin K to aid blood clotting and the application of eye ointment to prevent infections.

- **Initial feedings:** If the mother plans to breastfeed, the healthcare provider may assist with initiating breastfeeding or provide guidance on proper latching and positioning. The baby may receive the first bottle feeding if formula feeding is chosen.

- **Postnatal care and monitoring:** After the initial assessments and procedures, the baby is usually moved to the postnatal care area, where it will be monitored closely. This includes regular vital signs, feeding patterns, weight, and overall development checks.

Throughout this process, the healthcare team ensures the baby's comfort, monitors their well-being, and provides guidance and support to the parents. You and your partner need to engage with healthcare professionals, ask questions, and discuss any concerns you may have about your baby's health and care.

For a father and husband, your child's birth will be observed somewhat from the "sidelines." But as soon as the big day is over, you must offer support and anything else your wife and child need. Depending on the birthing process, your partner could be in a vulnerable and recovering state afterward. Be there for her in any way you can. It is essential to know what she is going through at those moments. Typically, the hospital stay for a vaginal birth is around 24 to 48 hours. In comparison, a C-section hospital stay usually ranges from 48 to 72 hours. Whichever path is taken, you and your new little family will return home soon!

Your partner will undoubtedly go through a period of physical and emotional recovery. Depending on the circumstances of the birth, your partner may experience physical discomfort, fatigue, and soreness. They may have postpartum bleeding, perineal pain (if there was tearing or an episiotomy), or breast engorgement if breastfeeding. They may have pain from birth or from stitches if they were required. Pain meds will help reduce the pain for your partner to rest. She may also experience fear with her first time peeing after birth. This is normal, so help her through the process and validate her feelings. She may also experience leakage as her pelvic floor is recovering from childbirth. This is also normal; you can support her with pregnancy pads or underwear. Overall, your partner needs to take time to rest, prioritize self-care, and allow her body to heal.

Moreover, the new baby can bring about a range of emotions for your partner. She may experience joy, excitement, and a deep sense of love for her newborn. However, she may also feel overwhelmed, anxious, or exhausted due to the demands of caring for a newborn and adjusting to her new role as a parent. All of these feelings are normal. Just remember to be there and offer reassurance, help, and motivation.

HOW TO A.C.E. THIS?!

Awareness:

Make sure you know the early signs of labor to help your partner time the contractions and know when to call your doctor so you can head to the hospital. Be aware of all the stages and processes during and after childbirth. Immediately after birth, and in those first few days afterward, your feelings of joy and excitement will intertwine with a lot of action, work, and learning new tasks. But one thing remains most important

- rest and recovery. These are crucial for the partner after the birth of their baby. And while much of the focus naturally goes toward the physical well-being of the person who gave birth, it's essential to recognize that the new father also needs time to heal and recharge. So always find time to be there for your partner and child, but also find a moment to recharge your batteries. It's a careful thing to balance out, but it's manageable.

Connection:

It goes without saying that it is vital for partners to communicate their needs for rest and recovery to their support network, whether it's family, friends, or healthcare professionals. Seeking help and accepting assistance with household chores, meal preparation, and other responsibilities allow both partners to focus on their well-being and bonding with their baby.

Remember, taking care of yourself is not selfish but rather a necessary step towards being the best support system for your partner. It also allows you to establish a strong bond with your baby. It provides you with opportunities for skin-to-skin contact, gentle cuddling, and engaging in soothing activities, all of which promote bonding and attachment. By caring for your own well-being, you can better engage with and connect with your newborn, fostering a nurturing and loving relationship.

Embrace:

People are very good at adapting to new situations and circumstances. In no time, you will find yourself boldly stepping into a new routine, a new life, and a new chapter. As you learn how to balance your new duties and find a bit of time for yourself, you will see that it is not all that difficult in the end. And before you know it, you will thrive in this brand new life - with your family! Take time to appreciate all the changes - big and small - you have made to improve yourself as a supportive partner and a first-time father. There's no feeling more incredible than this.

6

WELCOME HOME

B ringing a baby home is an exciting and transformative experience that marks the beginning of a new chapter in life. Numerous adjustments and changes await you as you embark on this parenthood journey. This chapter explores what to expect as you transition into life with a newborn, offering insights and guidance to help you navigate this precious and sometimes challenging time. Get ready to embrace the joys, challenges, and immense love that come with bringing your baby home.

Now, while it is true that the mother is most important to her baby in those first few days, your role will not be cast aside. In fact, after the baby's arrival, the father's role becomes exceptionally essential. But before we delve into all that, we must learn what happens in the hospital when the mother and child are ready to go home finally.

PREPARING FOR THE RIDE HOME

Typically, several key steps occur when a mother is ready to be discharged with her child. Here's what to expect:

- **Health Records and Birth Paperwork:** Before discharge, the hospital staff will provide you with health records and birth paperwork for your baby. This includes documents such as birth certificates, newborn screening results, and other relevant medical records. Make sure to review and keep these documents in a safe place, as they may be required for future appointments or administrative purposes.
- **Tests, Checks, and Vaccinations for Newborns:** Before leaving the hospital, your baby will undergo various tests and checks to ensure their well-being. This may include hearing screenings, blood tests, and physical examinations to assess their overall health. Additionally, your baby may receive necessary vaccinations according to the recommended immunization schedule. The healthcare team will inform you about these procedures and provide instructions or documentation regarding follow-up vaccinations or screenings.
- **Leaving the Hospital:** When it's time to leave the hospital, the healthcare team will provide you and your partner discharge instructions and guidance for caring for your baby at home. This may include information on feeding, bathing, diapering, and signs to watch out for that may indicate a need for medical attention. They

may also offer guidance on postpartum care for the birthing partner, including advice on pain management, wound care (if applicable for C-Sections), and emotional well-being.

Before leaving, it's essential to ensure you have all the necessities for your baby, such as appropriate clothing, blankets, diapers, and a properly installed car seat for safe transportation. The hospital staff may conduct a final check to ensure that your baby is securely placed in the car seat before you depart. Remember, don't hesitate to contact your healthcare provider or pediatrician if you have any questions or concerns during this transition. They are there to support you and guide you as you adjust to caring for your newborn at home.

And so, before you know it, your home is not just for you and your partner but also for your baby. As you get accustomed to the new setup, remember that the spotlight is equally on the three of you - your involvement counts as well! Your support is multifold and can always be appreciated. The postpartum period can bring a range of emotions for both parents. You play a vital role in offering emotional support and understanding to your partner. In fact, you can provide a listening ear, offer reassurance, and validate your partner's experiences and feelings. This support helps create a nurturing and comforting environment, enabling the birthing partner to navigate the emotional ups and downs of early parenthood with greater ease. And it also lays down the foundations of a healthy and happy family.

SHARE THE RESPONSIBILITIES

Of course, it would be wrong not to involve yourself with the activities around the baby - activities that are naturally and traditionally given to women. Contrary to popular belief, fathers can establish a deep bond with their babies from the beginning. They can engage in activities such as holding, soothing, and feeding (if bottle-feeding) the baby. This active involvement fosters a sense of connection, love, and responsibility, strengthening the parent-child relationship. So, you see that your presence and engagement in caregiving tasks also provide your wife with much-needed respite and support. Break those aged stereotypes that state how men should not be involved in functions related to the baby, and take matters into your own hands. It's time that men show that they can be loving fathers, caring husbands, and strong providers.

But at the same time, remember that parenthood is a shared journey, and your involvement as a father allows for a more balanced distribution of responsibilities. You can take on tasks such as diaper changes, bathing, comforting the baby, and assisting with household chores. By actively participating in caring for the baby, you help create a supportive and nurturing environment for the entire family. But in the end, you need to communicate openly with your partner about your desires, concerns, and limitations - and vice versa. Each family's dynamics and needs are unique, so finding a balance that works for both partners is vital. With clear and open communication, progress and happiness are achievable.

Being a parent is a beautiful thing. It is one of nature's awe-inspiring miracles. Just think about it: you have created this tiny human, a new life that blooms and develops before your very eyes. Words cannot describe the feeling - the concept itself.

But a lot of it is a mystery as well. You must understand what happens to your child and how the baby develops in those first few weeks and months.

WHAT TO EXPECT IN YOUR BABY'S FIRST MONTH

Even though it might not seem so, newborns lose a small amount of weight in the first month before gaining and growing in length. Your baby should regain that weight in their first two weeks. They gradually develop more control over their movements, although their actions may still appear jerky and uncoordinated. Newborns are highly responsive to sensory stimuli. They can see objects and people at close distances, but their vision is still blurry. Babies are attracted to bright colors and high-contrast patterns. They also have a strong sense of hearing and can recognize familiar voices, often turning their heads toward sounds. And while newborns may seem primarily focused on meeting their immediate needs, they are beginning to develop early cognitive skills. They can recognize their caregivers' faces and respond to soothing sounds or voices. They may also start displaying brief moments of alertness and curiosity about their surroundings.

Unsurprisingly, babies in their first month communicate primarily through crying, facial expressions, and body movements. They rely on caregivers to meet their needs for feeding, diaper changes, and comfort. They begin to establish a bond with their primary caregivers and show a preference for familiar faces. Don't be annoyed or unsettled by your baby's crying - most of the time, it's just their way of expressing a need. As a father, you must learn patience and understanding, even if you sometimes don't feel you could.

Newborns sleep often, typically around 16-17 hours a day, although their sleep is fragmented into shorter periods. They have irregular sleep patterns, alternating between deep sleep and periods of wakefulness. Use the time when they sleep to focus on your activities or something that needs to be done around the home.

It's important to note that each baby develops at their own pace, and there may be variations in individual growth and milestones. Monitoring your baby's growth, observing their responses, and engaging in interactive activities such as talking, singing, and applying gentle touch can support their development during this crucial first month of life.

WHAT TO EXPECT IN YOUR BABY'S SECOND MONTH

As you begin a life alongside your baby, you will notice how quickly time passes and how they develop even faster. Changes can appear literally overnight. In the second month, your baby will make significant developmental strides. Babies in the second month start to gain more control over their movements. They can hold their heads up briefly while lying on their stomachs and may even lift their chest during tummy time. Their movements become less jerky and more purposeful. They may also begin to bring their hands to their mouth and grasp objects intentionally. Visual abilities improve during the second month. Babies can track objects with their eyes and focus on faces or toys. They become more responsive to visual stimuli and can distinguish between different shapes and patterns. Their hearing continues to develop, and they may turn their heads toward familiar sounds and voices. Babies begin to make a variety of sounds during the second month. They coo, gurgle, and make babbling sounds. They may start to respond to their caregivers' voices by cooing back or attempting to imitate sounds. They may also exhibit different cries for various needs, such as hunger, discomfort, or tiredness.

And - *something parents love hearing* - babies start to develop more consistent sleep patterns by the second month, with longer stretches of sleep at night. However, they may still wake up for feeding or diaper changes. Establishing a routine and creating a sleep-friendly environment can promote more regular sleep patterns for everyone.

Remember, each baby develops at their own pace, so what goes for other babies might not be true for yours.

HOW TO A.C.E. BEING A DAD!

When it comes to being a dad, utilizing the A.C.E. method (Awareness, Connection, Embrace) is crucial for building a strong bond with your baby and supporting your partner during the postpartum period. One of the critical aspects of this method is taking advantage of parental leaves and actively participating in caring for your baby while your partner recovers. Taking as much time off work as possible will be incredibly rewarding to your partner, your newborn, and you. In this next section, you will learn many tasks that will help you excel in all three areas of the A.C.E. method to bond with your newborn. Here are various tips and step-by-step guides to help you navigate this new journey:

- **Educate Yourself:** Familiarize yourself with baby care essentials by reading books, attending parenting classes, or seeking guidance from healthcare professionals. Learn about feeding, diapering, bathing, and soothing techniques. Understanding your baby's needs and milestones will boost your confidence in caring for them.
- **Communicate and Collaborate:** Open communication with your partner is vital. Discuss your roles and responsibilities, expectations, and concerns. Collaborate on caregiving tasks, including feeding, changing diapers, and putting the baby to sleep. Sharing the duties strengthens your bond as parents and promotes an equal partnership.
- **Bonding Time:** Spend quality time bonding with your baby. Engage in activities like cuddling, singing, talking, and playing. You can perform skin-to-skin contact by holding your baby against your bare chest, which promotes bonding and helps regulate their temperature and heart rate.
- **Learn Baby Cues:** Observe your baby's cues and respond to their needs promptly. Learn to distinguish

hunger, tiredness, discomfort, and other signals.
Respond affectionately, meet their needs, and comfort
them when upset. Developing sensitivity to your baby's
cues strengthens your connection and builds trust.

- **Maintain Self-Care:** Remember to prioritize your own
well-being. Take breaks, engage in hobbies, exercise,
and find ways to rest and recharge your batteries.
Taking care of yourself allows you to be present and
better equipped to care for your baby and support your
partner.

- **Seek Help:** Don't hesitate to ask for help when needed.
Reach out to family, friends, or professional support if
you feel overwhelmed or need guidance. Parenting is a
learning process, and seeking assistance along the way
is okay. The others know this too and won't hesitate to
help when possible.

Of course, as an able and involved father, you must also learn
how to care for the baby and its various needs. The tasks you
need to know how to perform include swaddling, calming,
feeding, and many others. After all, sometimes you will find
yourself alone with your newborn. You will have to know how
to take care of things. Here's a quick rundown of essential skills
you should learn to become a confident, super dad:

Holding Your Baby:

- **Cradle Hold:** Place one arm under the baby's head and neck. Their head should be lying in the crook or bend of your arm. Place your other arm around their bottom. Keep their head supported and close to your chest.
- **Football Hold:** Position the baby's head in the palm of your hand, facing your side. Use your arm to support their back and bottom. This is a typical position mom may use for breastfeeding. However, you can also perform this hold with one side of your baby's face in the palm of your hand. Their belly will rest on your arm while their arms and legs dangle downward. Whichever way you face your baby, it should feel like you're holding a football. Just don't fumble this one.
- **Over-the-Shoulder Hold:** Bring your baby's face gently to lean onto one shoulder. With the arm of the same shoulder your baby is on, support your baby's bottom. Place your other hand on their back and neck to keep them supported and leaning onto your shoulder.
- Always, always, always ensure that your baby's head and neck are supported, as they have not developed any neck strength at these early stages of life. Avoid sudden movements as well.

Feeding Your Baby:

- Prepare your bottle. If you and your partner are exclusively breastfeeding, take a 2-ounce bottle from her supply. Breast milk can be stored for up to 4 hours, unrefrigerated, or refrigerated for up to 4 days. If you are using formula, follow the instructions carefully for mixing formula with water. Do your best not to water it down or make it too concentrated, as this can disturb your baby's electrolytes. Find the right bottle, as bottles have various nipple shapes. Your baby may like a particular shape, and that will improve both of your feeding experiences. Use a slow-flow nipple to mimic breastfeeding.
- Use a bottle warmer to warm up the milk. You can also place the bottle in a container or basin of warm water to heat it up. Test the temperature of the milk by squeezing a few drops onto your skin before feeding.
- Place your baby in the cradle position. Try to have them at a 45-degree angle so that their head is propped up.
- Feed your baby the warm milk. Newborns typically consume 1-2 ounces of milk every 2-3 hours. You will know when they are done eating as they will spit up more or lose interest in sucking the bottle. This is your time to learn your baby's feeding schedule, which will help you know what to expect, especially at night.
- Burp your baby when they are done feeding. Put a towel on your shoulder to prevent a mess if your baby spits milk. Place your baby in the over-the-shoulder position. Pat their back gently until they burp. This may

take a couple of minutes. Burping is essential as feeding causes more air intake than when your baby usually breathes, which can lead to gas and fussiness.

Swaddling Your Baby:

- Lay a blanket flat on a safe surface in a diamond shape.
- Fold down the top corner to create a straight edge, and place the baby's head above the fold.
- Place the baby's arms alongside their body and snugly wrap one side of the blanket across their chest.
- Fold the bottom corner up and tuck it under the first fold.
- Finally, wrap the remaining side of the blanket across the baby's chest and tuck it securely.

Calming Your Baby:

- Create a soothing environment by dimming lights, playing soft music, or using white noise, such as running a gentle fan.
- Hold your baby close to your chest and gently rock them in your arms or a rocking chair.
- Use soft, rhythmic shushing sounds or gentle humming to comfort the baby. Try singing to them softly. It's okay; you don't have to be a good singer.
- Offer a pacifier or allow them to suck on a clean finger. This provides a sense of comfort for them.
- Try gentle infant massage or provide gentle, rhythmic strokes on their back or tummy. All three of my kids

were easily soothed with delicate ear and temple massages. Every baby is different, so you'll have to do some trial and error to find out what they like best.

- Sometimes they may be crying and fussy from gas. Try burping them. You can also place them on a comfortable surface in a laying or sitting position. Hold each ankle with both hands and move their legs as if they are riding a bicycle. This can encourage your baby to pass gas and even poop. They may have just needed that relief!

Changing Their Diaper:

- Gather all the necessary supplies before beginning. You'll need clean diapers, baby wipes or a washcloth, diaper rash cream (if needed), and a changing pad or a clean, soft surface.
- Find a safe and comfortable space for diaper changing. Lay down a changing pad or spread out a clean towel or blanket.
- Unfasten the diaper tabs by removing any adhesive straps. Carefully lift the baby's bottom off the diaper, and fold the front of the dirty diaper down. Use the clean front part of the diaper to wipe away any excess waste.
- Grab a baby wipe or a damp washcloth and gently clean the baby's diaper area, starting from the front (for girls) or top (for boys) and wiping toward the back. Be sure to clean all the creases and folds, including the genital area and buttocks. You may want to use warm water and a

washcloth instead of cold wipes for newborns, as their skin is delicate and unable to regulate temperature. Remember to always wipe from front to back as you don't want to get their poop into the genital areas.

- Remove the dirty diaper from under your baby's bottom by gently lifting them by their legs.
- Apply diaper rash cream or baby powder (if needed).
- Open a clean diaper and slide it under the baby, positioning the back half of the diaper under their bottom. Bring the front part up between the baby's legs. Fasten the diaper snugly using the adhesive tabs. Try to make sure the diaper is not too tight so you don't damage your baby's delicate skin.

Bathing Your Baby:

- Gather all necessary supplies: a baby bathtub or basin, mild baby soap, a soft washcloth, towels, and clean clothes.
- Fill the tub with a few inches of warm water (around 37°C or 98.6°F).
- Test the water temperature with your elbow or a thermometer to ensure it's not too hot.
- Support your baby's head and neck with one hand and slowly lower them into the water, using your other hand to guide their body.
- Use a gentle touch to wash their body, starting with their face, then moving to their arms and legs. Use mild soap sparingly and avoid getting water in their eyes or ears.

- Rinse your baby with a clean, damp washcloth or gently pour warm water over their body.
- Lift your baby out of the tub and wrap them in a warm towel, patting them dry.
- Dress them in clean clothes and ensure they are comfortable and warm.
- Remember, safety is paramount when handling a baby. Always support their head and neck, ensure appropriate water temperature, and never leave them unattended during bathing.

Putting Your Baby to Sleep:

You will perform many of the actions recommended in the calming section, but here are more tips for excellent sleep hygiene.

- Gently rock them in your arms or while holding them in a rocking chair to soothe them to sleep. Massage their belly, back, ears or feet to comfort them. Swaddling can help prevent your baby from jerky movements that may wake them up.
- Carefully lay them in their crib after they fall asleep in your arms. Mastering this transition will allow you to complete other tasks your partner may need help with, like cleaning the house, preparing food, or other first-time dad duties.
- Get blackout curtains. This will make the room dark and stimulant-free, which is a benefit for your baby and

for you and your partner to take much-needed naps
during the day.

- Use white noise, such as a fan to soft music, to keep
  them asleep while you get in and out of bed, enter and
  exit the room, and complete household chores.
- Another essential tip is to change your baby's diaper
  before bedtime. This will prevent you from changing
  their diaper more than needed during the night. Doing
  this lets you feed your baby at night and put them back
  to sleep with ease. Changing diapers at night will wake
  them up, and you will have to start the calming and
  sleeping process again.

Practice these skills with care and patience, and soon your
confidence in caring for your little one will be through the roof.

HOW TO A.C.E. BEING A PARTNER!

Being a caring dad, attentive husband, and responsible adult is
absolutely challenging. Finding the right balance between all
three takes a lot of work. But that doesn't mean you can't A.C.E.
it and do it in style. You *can*, and you *will* stay on top of things
and proudly carry the new parenthood era of your life on your
shoulders. And this involves not just being a great dad but also
a great partner. So how do you A.C.E. being a partner at the
same time you're acing fatherhood? Here are some tips to help
you stay on top:

Awareness:

Parenthood is a shared responsibility. Nobody is alone in this. Parenthood is a team effort. Divide duties with your partner to alleviate the workload. Be actively involved in caregiving tasks, such as feeding, diaper changes, soothing the baby, and household chores. Taking turns waking up at night to feed and change your baby is a great thing to do. Working together creates a sense of partnership and reduces the burden on one person.

Realize that your new life will get busy, so do your best to stay organized and on top of things. An organized mind is a successful mind. Don't get lost in the chaos of each day and ultimately lose control of everything. Instead, manage your time and responsibilities more effectively. Use tools like calendars, to-do lists, or mobile apps to stay on top of appointments, baby milestones, and household tasks. Planning ahead can reduce stress and ensure you're both prepared for the day-to-day challenges. Your partner will definitely appreciate an orderly, organized, and in-control male counterpart.

Remember that you need to take time for yourself. People are not made of stone. The pressure of daily life needs to be released somehow. That is why caring for yourself is essential to support your partner better. Prioritize self-care activities, such as getting enough rest, eating nutritious meals, and engaging in activities you enjoy. Do hobbies and things that you love. Even an hour per day can be enough to recharge your batteries. My best advice concerning self-care is to take naps or sleep when your baby is sleeping. Your baby will likely keep you and your partner up at night with feedings every 2-3 hours, so you will both lack a lot of sleep. Sleeping when your baby sleeps will help you replenish your energy levels to ensure you can be the best partner and father you strive to be.

Connection:

Show that you care by regularly expressing your love and appreciation for your partner. Small gestures like saying "thank you," giving compliments, and offering hugs and kisses can go a long way in strengthening your bond. Recognize and acknowledge your partner's efforts in parenting and maintaining the household. Be happy in your new life - it will get you further, faster.

Nurture your relationship by keeping your romance alive. It's foolish to say that a newborn will *"extinguish"* the romance and passion in a relationship. Even when it's tough, you need to keep the romance alive. So set aside quality time for just the two of you, even if it's just a few minutes each day. Plan date nights, take walks together, or enjoy a quiet evening at home. Keep the romance alive by expressing your love and affection for each other. And yes, I know what you're thinking. When can you and your partner have sex again?! Most doctors recommend waiting four to six weeks after having a baby. This waiting period allows your partner's uterus to return to normal. Be patient with her and find a time that is right for both of you to resume intimacy.

Embrace:

Remember, parenthood is a learning process. Life itself is one continuous learning process. The world does not demand that you ace everything all at once and excel in all spheres of life by default. No - you will have to learn that, take things one step at a time, and embrace the quirky chaos of family life. But throughout that learning process, you will discover endless love, joy, fun, passion, confidence, and strength. And that's what matters at the end of the day. That's what will fill your heart!

So don't close your mind, don't close your heart, and don't shy away from a new challenge. Be open - let the new experiences flood your senses and provide you with the necessary arsenal to conquer all of life's challenging milestones. With each new day, you become a stronger, better, and more confident version of yourself. And the world will know it.

7

_____

WHAT ABOUT DAD?

Even if it's the 21st century, and we are boldly stepping towards new standards and open minds, many ancient misconceptions surround parenthood. They come from an age of fixed gender roles and many incorrect worldviews. These are the views of our great-grandfathers, of stern men dictated by their times' norms. But these times are different. This is a time when _we_ create an environment in which we want to live. This entire book aims to break these outdated gender roles and offer a fresh, bold, and completely normal outlook on fatherhood. Fathers often find themselves overlooked unjustly in discussions surrounding parenthood, and it's essential to recognize their significant role. While the focus is rightly placed on mothers during pregnancy, childbirth, and the early stages of parenting, first-time dads also play a crucial part in the journey. They provide love and support to their partners and children, and their involvement is essential for the overall well-being of the family unit. Fathers deserve recognition for their dedication, sacrifices, and contributions to raising their children. We need to create a society that values and acknowledges the role of fathers, promoting equal parenting partnerships and encouraging their active involvement in all aspects of their child's life. That topic also touches upon gender equality, shared parenthood roles, traditional values, and a healthy family. So, in this final chapter, we ask ourselves: *"What about Dad?"*

You are important too! You must always keep this in mind, especially when handling everything that gets tough. Whatever you face, and no matter how hard - you are significant. Let that be the guiding light toward ultimate success. But it can be challenging. It *will* be challenging. That's no secret.

Sometimes, the burdens can seem overwhelming, and depression can take hold. That's right - postpartum depression is not limited only to mothers. New dads can also experience this state, which is often referred to as *paternal postpartum depression (P.P.D.)*. This condition can manifest in various ways, including feelings of sadness, anxiety, irritability, and a loss of interest in activities. To keep P.P.D. at bay, we must emphasize the significance of caring for one's overall well-being as a new dad. Familiarize yourself with the signs and symptoms of paternal postpartum depression. These can include persistent feelings of sadness or emptiness, changes in appetite or sleep patterns, difficulty concentrating, loss of interest, irritability, and withdrawal from family and friends. If you notice these symptoms persisting for an extended period, seeking support and professional help is essential. Don't hesitate to seek support from your partner, family, friends, or healthcare professionals. Discuss your feelings and concerns openly, and don't try to handle everything alone. Sharing your experiences and seeking assistance can help alleviate the burden and provide valuable insights and guidance.

Taking care of yourself is crucial for your overall well-being. Make self-care a priority by engaging in activities that bring you joy and relaxation. This can include exercise, hobbies, spending time with friends, or pursuing personal interests. Taking breaks and having time for yourself allows you to recharge and better support your partner and baby.

Only as you recognize that you are *needed and appreciated* and have a critical role to commit to will you be able to be at your happiest and most fulfilled. So, *what about Dad? Dad is right there, and he* **matters.**

Your role during pregnancy is essential in supporting and nurturing both your partner and your growing baby. It is so important and has many facets. A father's support is material, physical, and emotional. Undoubtedly, a father's support towards the mother is significant. The involvement of dads has numerous benefits for a mother's overall well-being. It fosters a sense of emotional support, reduces stress, and promotes a positive mental and emotional state. Mothers who feel supported and understood by their partners are more likely to have a smoother transition into motherhood and experience fewer instances of postpartum depression or anxiety.

Additionally, a father's active involvement in parenting promotes bonding between the father and the child. It allows for the development of a robust father-child relationship from the early stages, which is crucial for the child's emotional and social development.

Parenthood is a transformative journey that defies preparation. Despite all the efforts made to plan, learn, and gather knowledge, no one can ever fully prepare for the experience of becoming a parent. Parenthood brings unique challenges, joys, and surprises that are impossible to predict or fully understand until one embarks on the journey. Each child is special, and every parent-child relationship unfolds in its own way. Parents learn and grow alongside their children through lived experiences, trial and error, and unconditional love. Parenthood is a constant learning process, requiring adaptability, patience, and an open heart. Embracing the unpredictable nature of parenthood allows for the discovery of profound moments of connection, growth, and the unbreakable bond between parent and child. So never give up. Stay committed, stay positive, stay confident. This is a lifetime journey, and being a part of it is so amazing!

HOW TO A.C.E. YOUR NEW ROLE

To the last, we stick firmly to the A.C.E. method. It is a straightforward cornerstone towards guaranteed success. Following it, you can be sure to maintain a focus at all times, keeping your goal and your motivations affixed in front of you - an end result you'll always strive to reach. It was with us from page one and can be efficiently applied to any sphere of pregnancy and early fatherhood.

So, in these finalizing pages of our book - our shared learning journey - we once more focus on the A.C.E. method. This time, it becomes our final mantra, a summary of all the steps we've taken thus far.

Awareness:

Gaining awareness of stressors and knowing when to step back and recollect oneself is crucial for maintaining emotional well-being as a parent. Engage in mindfulness exercises such as deep breathing, meditation, or body scans. These practices help you tune into your emotions, thoughts, and physical sensations, allowing you to recognize signs of stress and take appropriate action.

Take time to journal and reflect on your experiences, emotions, and challenges. Writing can help you gain clarity, process emotions, and identify patterns or triggers that contribute to stress. Furthermore, recognize your limits and set boundaries to protect your well-being. Learn to say no when necessary, delegate tasks, and prioritize self-care to prevent burnout. You should also pay attention to physical and emotional signs of stress, such as tension, fatigue, irritability, or changes in appetite or sleep patterns. When these signs arise, take it as a cue to step back, take a break, and engage in self-care strategies to recalibrate. Remember, awareness of your personal state is paramount - without that awareness, you can't be the ideal partner and father you strive to be.

Connection:

Connecting with people can significantly lessen stress and anxiety for expectant dads. They can find support, gain perspective, and navigate their roles by engaging with their partner, friends, and families. First and foremost, you should connect with your partner. Connecting with your partner allows you to share your worries, fears, and excitement about becoming a parent. By communicating openly and actively listening, partners can provide emotional support, problem-solve together, and strengthen their relationship.

Of course, maintaining connections with friends who have experienced parenthood or are going through a similar phase can be invaluable. Sharing experiences, seeking advice, and simply having someone to talk to helps provide camaraderie and reassurance. Friends can offer practical tips, lend an empathetic ear, or even provide a much-needed break from parental responsibilities. Lastly, joining parenting communities or support groups can connect dads-to-be with others in a similar life phase. These communities offer a platform to share experiences, seek advice, and learn from one another. Building relationships within these communities fosters a sense of belonging, reduces isolation, and provides a valuable support network. You can even make strong friendships that will last a lifetime!

Embrace:

Changes are not to be shunned; they are to be *embraced*. Embrace what life gives you, and you will turn out stronger and better as a result. Embracing fatherhood brings numerous benefits to you, your partner, and your child in the long run. It creates a stronger bond with both your partner and your child. Actively participating in caregiving, playing, and spending quality time together strengthens emotional connections and creates lifelong memories. By embracing fatherhood, you become a positive role model for your child. Remember that fathers teach fundamental values, provide guidance, and demonstrate healthy relationship dynamics, which sets a foundation for every child's development and future relationships. Overall, embracing fatherhood will positively impact your child's social, emotional, and cognitive development. Active engagement in play, communication, and learning activities stimulates their growth, enhances their self-esteem, and fosters their overall development.

Remember, no one becomes a perfect father overnight. It's a learning process, and you have already shown your commitment by seeking knowledge and guidance. Trust in your ability to adapt, grow, and make the best decisions for yourself, your partner, and your child. As you embark on this incredible journey, embrace the lessons you have learned from this book and apply them in your everyday life. Take comfort in knowing that you have equipped yourself with valuable tools to face the joys and challenges of pregnancy and fatherhood. Approach each day with optimism, patience, and an open heart. Be present, actively engage with your partner and child, and cherish the precious moments you will share together. Remember to take care of yourself, seek support when needed, and be patient with yourself as you learn and grow. It is vital to believe in your abilities, to be humble and patient, kind and forgiving. Understanding is mandatory in parenthood, as is love and happiness.

You have what it takes to A.C.E. your new roles as a supportive and confident first-time father: be Aware, Communicate openly, and Embrace the joys and challenges. Trust in your instincts, love unconditionally and create a nurturing environment for your growing family. The rest? The rest comes naturally.

WHETHER YOUR NEWBORN HAS ARRIVED OR YOU ARE STILL WAITING, KEEP ACEING IT!

It's great that you have taken this step to become a better partner and father. All the research supports the benefits of dad's involvement early on and you are making sure your newborn has the best start in life. How about giving other children the same opportunity?

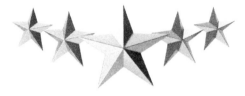

LEAVE A REVIEW!

Your opinions matter so much. Remember how you were feeling at the beginning of this book compared to now? Think about how your relationship has changed for the better. In just a couple of minutes, you could do the same for another couple! Thank you so much and have fun in your new role— there is none other like it!

Scan the QR codes for a quick review!

CONCLUSION

And so we reach the last pages of our written adventure. With the knowledge and confidence gained from this book, you are ready to embark on this incredible journey of pregnancy and early fatherhood. Embrace the experience, enjoy the moments, and create a lifetime of beautiful memories with your partner and your newborn. Happiness is *not* one step away - happiness has *already begun.*

Throughout this book, you've gained essential knowledge, practical tips, and heartfelt insights to prepare you for the incredible role of fatherhood. The key takeaway from our shared journey is that you have the power to be an exceptional partner and a confident first-time dad. Each chapter has equipped you with valuable tools to navigate the challenges, celebrate the joys, and create a loving environment for your growing family. By embracing the lessons learned here, you can overcome self-doubt and fears, allowing your confidence to shine. Remember, you are not alone in this journey. Countless dads have successfully embraced fatherhood, and so can you. Now, it's time to put your newfound knowledge into action. Embrace the ups and downs, trust your instincts, and be present for every milestone.

Please take the opportunity to leave a positive review of this book on Amazon and share your experience. By taking a few seconds to do this, you will help other dads find the support and guidance they need.

As the author of this book, I assure you that you have what it takes to be a fantastic partner and first-time father. Embrace this exciting chapter in your life, knowing you are equipped with the tools, love, and determination to create a beautiful family story. You can also be glad to know that all the information presented here comes from an experienced father. I've crossed the path you are traversing and bore the challenges you now bear. Let that be the reassurance you need and a helping hand from one father to another. After all, would success be possible without teamwork?

In the end, thank you for embarking on this journey with me. I hope you enjoyed learning from my experiences and insight as much as I loved sharing them with you. May you thrive, grow, and create cherished memories as you become the greatest partner and first-time father you can be. You *got this!*

REFERENCES

10 Popular Quotes About Fatherhood. (2022, June 9). https://story.motherhood. com.my/blog/10-popular-quotes-about-fatherhood/

American Pregnancy Association. (2023). *Knowing Baby's Sex Before Birth: Some Pros and Cons of Gender Reveal.* Retrieved from https://americanpreg nancy.org/healthy-pregnancy/pregnancy-products-tests/knowing-babys-sex-before-birth-some-pros-and-cons-of-gender-reveal/

Beairsto, R. (2020, September 29). *How to Choose a Pediatrician for Your New Baby. Healthline.* Retrieved from https://www.healthline.com/health/chil drens-health/how-to-choose-a-pediatrician

BetterHealth Victoria. (2023, March 16). *First Days After Birth. Better Health.* Retrieved from https://www.betterhealth.vic.gov.au/health/servicesand support/first-days-after-birth

Beyond Blue. (2022). *Adjusting to Parenthood.* Beyond Blue. Retrieved from https://healthyfamilies.beyondblue.org.au/pregnancy-and-new-parents/ becoming-a-parent-what-to-expect/adjusting-to-parenthood

Birth Injury Help Center. (2023). *Pregnancy Complications.* Birthing Injury Help Center. Retrieved from https://birthinjuryhelpcenter.org/complica tion-pregnant.html

Brookwood Women's Medical Center. (n.d.). *5 Tips to Ease New Dad Fears.* Retrieved from https://www.brookwoodwomensmedicalcenter.com/ stories/stories/5-tips-to-ease-new-dad-fears

Chertoff, J. (2018, November 29). *How to Bathe a Newborn Baby: A Step-by-Step Guide. Healthline.* Retrieved from https://www.healthline.com/health/ parenting/how-to-bathe-newborn

Cleveland Clinic. (2023). *Pregnancy: Second Trimester.* Retrieved from https:// my.clevelandclinic.org/health/articles/16092-pregnancy-second-trimester

Geddes, J. (2021. January 6). *How to Soothe a Crying Baby.* What to Expect. Retrieved from https://www.whattoexpect.com/first-year/care/how-to-make-baby-stop-crying

Graves, G. (2020. July 22). How to Create Your Birth Plan: *A Checklist for*

Parents. Parents. Retrieved from https://www.parents.com/pregnancy/giving-birth/labor-and-delivery/checklist-how-to-write-a-birth-plan/

Hello Postpartum. (2022, October 17). *How to Support Your Pregnant Wife.* Retrieved from https://hellopostpartum.com/how-to-support-your-pregnant-wife/

Higuera, V. (2020. June 18). *7 Things to Consider When Choosing a Pediatrician.* Healthline. Retrieved from https://www.healthline.com/health/childrens-health/how-to-choose-a-pediatrician

Hopkins Medicine. (2023). *The Second Trimester of Pregnancy: What to Expect.* Retrieved from https://www.hopkinsmedicine.org/health/wellness-and-prevention/the-second-trimester

Jones-Choi, A. (2022. March 4). *12 Tips for When Dad Feeds a Newborn.* Mom. Retrieved from https://mom.com/baby/12-tips-for-when-dad-feeds-a-newborn

Kahn, A. (2018, December 3). *Second Trimester Complications and How to Handle Them. Healthline.* Retrieved from https://www.healthline.com/health/pregnancy/second-trimester-complications

Killian, J (2023). *How to Embrace Fatherhood.* Arcadian Counseling. Retrieved from https://arcadiancounseling.com/how-to-embrace-fatherhood/

Marcin, A. (2020. September 10). *Getting Ready for the Big Day: Packing Your Hospital Bag.* Healthline. Retrieved from https://www.healthline.com/health/pregnancy/hospital-bag-checklist

March of Dimes. (2018). *Your Body After Baby: The First 6 Weeks.* Retrieved from https://marchofdimes.org/find-support/topics/postpartum/your-body-after-baby-first-6-weeks

Mauer, E. (2017. May 17). *What Happens at the Hospital When You Deliver.* The Bump. Retrieved from https://www.thebump.com/a/what-to-expect-at-the-hospital-during-labor

Mayo Clinic. (2022, April 27). *Infant and toddler health.* Retrieved from https://www.mayoclinic.org/healthy-lifestyle/infant-and-toddler-health/in-depth/healthy-baby/art-20047741

Mayo Clinic. (2022, July 27). *Overdue Pregnancy: What to Do When Baby's Past Due.* Retrieved from https://www.mayoclinic.org/healthy-lifestyle/pregnancy-week-by-week/in-depth/overdue-pregnancy/art-20048287

Mayo Clinic. (2022, December 6). *Postpartum Care: What to Expect After a Vaginal Delivery.* Retrieved from https://www.mayoclinic.org/healthy-lifestyle/labor-and-delivery/in-depth/postpartum-care/art-20047233

Medical News Today. (2019, February 22). *What to know about sex during pregnancy.* Retrieved from https://www.medicalnewstoday.com/articles/321648#benefits

Mental Health America. (2023). *Mental Health and New Father.* Retrieved from https://mhanational.org/mental-health-and-new-father

NCT. (2017). *First Trimester Tips for Dads-to-Be.* Retrieved from https://www.nct.org.uk/pregnancy/dads-be/first-trimester-tips-for-dads-be

National Health Service. (2020, November 12). *Antenatal Classes.* Retrieved from https://www.nhs.uk/pregnancy/your-pregnancy-care/your-antenatal-care/

National Health Service. (2020, November 30). *What Happens at the Hospital or Birth Centre.* Retrieved from https://www.nhs.uk/pregnancy/labour-and-birth/signs-of-labour/what-happens-at-the-hospital-or-birth-centre/

National Health Service. (2022, August 22). *What Happens Straight After the Birth?* Retrieved from https://www.nhs.uk/pregnancy/labour-and-birth/after-the-birth/what-happens-straight-after/

National Childbirth Trust (2017, March). *Dad-to-be Guide: 10 Facts for the Third Trimester.* Retrieved from https://www.nct.org.uk/pregnancy/dads-be/dad-be-guide-10-facts-for-third-trimester

National Institute Child Health and Human Development. (2018. November 6). *What are some factors that make a pregnancy high risk?* Retrieved from https://www.nichd.nih.gov/health/topics/high-risk/conditioninfo/factors

New America. (n.d.). *What Are the Biggest Challenges Fathers Face?* Retrieved from https://www.newamerica.org/better-life-lab/reports/engaged-dads-and-opportunities-and-barriers-equal-parenting-united-states/what-are-the-biggest-challenges-fathers-face/

Pampers. (2020. September 6). *How to Swaddle Your Baby.* Retrieved from https://www.pampers.com/en-us/baby/sleep/article/how-to-swaddle-a-baby

Parker, W. (2022. October 5). *How to Help Your Partner Through the Last Month of Pregnancy.* Verywell Family Retrieved from https://www.verywellfamily.com/making-it-through-last-pregnancy-month-1270769

Planned Parenthood (2023). *What happens in the fourth month of pregnancy.* Retrieved from https://www.plannedparenthood.org/learn/pregnancy/pregnancy-month-by-month/what-happens-fourth-month-pregnancy

Planned Parenthood (2023). *What happens in the fifth month of pregnancy.*

Retrieved from https://www.plannedparenthood.org/learn/pregnancy/pregnancy-month-by-month/what-happens-fourth-month-pregnancy https://www.plannedparenthood.org/learn/pregnancy/pregnancy-month-by-month/what-happens-fifth-month-pregnancy

Planned Parenthood (2023). *What happens in the sixth month of pregnancy.* Retrieved from https://www.plannedparenthood.org/learn/pregnancy/pregnancy-month-by-month/what-happens-sixth-month-pregnancy

Planned Parenthood (2023). *What happens in the seventh month of pregnancy.* Retrieved from https://www.plannedparenthood.org/learn/pregnancy/pregnancy-month-by-month/what-happens-seventh-month-pregnancy

Planned Parenthood (2023). *What happens in the eighth month of pregnancy.* Retrieved from https://www.plannedparenthood.org/learn/pregnancy/pregnancy-month-by-month/what-happens-eighth-month-pregnancy

PsychCentral. (2023). *Tips to Help Reconnect with Your Partner After Baby.* Retrieved from https://psychcentral.com/relationships/tips-to-help-reconnect-with-your-partner-after-baby

Raising Children (2023. March 5). *How to hold a newborn: in pictures.* Retrieved from https://raisingchildren.net.au/newborns/health-daily-care/holding-newborns/how-to-hold-your-newborn

Rockliffe, L. (2023. March 10). *The importance of social support in pregnancy and ways to connect with others.* Tommy. Retrieved from https://www.tommys.org/pregnancy-information/pregnancy-news-blogs/pregnancy-news-blogs-being-pregnant/importance-social-support

Stanford Medicine Children's Health. (2023). *Care of the Baby in the Delivery Room.* Retrieved from https://www.stanfordchildrens.org/en/topic/default?id=care-of-the-baby-in-the-delivery-room-90-P02871

Tommy's. (2022. June 16). *Supporting your partner's mental health.* Retrieved from https://www.tommys.org/pregnancy-information/dads-and-partners/your-partners-mental-health-after-the-birth

Tommy's. (2023. July 6). *Antenatal classes - preparing you for birth.* Retrieved from https://www.tommys.org/pregnancy-information/im-pregnant/antenatal-care/antenatal-classes-preparing-you-birth

Tommys. (2019, December 18). *Your relationship with your partner after a miscarriage.* Retrieved from https://www.tommys.org/baby-loss-support/miscarriage-information-and-support/support-after-miscarriage/your-relationship-your-partner-after-miscarriage

WebMD Archives. (n.d.). *Getting Pregnant Can Be Harder Than It Looks.*

WebMD. Retrieved from https://www.webmd.com/infertility-and-repro duction/features/getting-pregnant-can-be-harder-than-looks

Wilson, C. (2016). *First Baby Stress in New Dads.* Focus on the Family. Retrieved from https://www.focusonthefamily.ca/content/first-baby-stress-in-new-dads

Wisner, W. (2012, August 12). *Your 3-Month-Old Baby's Milestones & Development.* Verywell Family. Retrieved from https://www.verywellfam ily.com/your-3-month-old-baby-development-and-milestones-4172049

Printed in Great Britain
by Amazon

37097248R00089